DEATH BY DIET

This publication is intended to direct the attention of both physician and patient to the torrent of scientific research being carried out on the significance of biological calcium. It is for educational purposes. It is not intended to replace the orthodox physician-patient relationship. If you are sick, you are advised to consult a physician, and together, along with your newly gained knowledge, work towards the resolution of your illness.

Robert R. Barefoot

i

DEATH BY DIET

By

Robert R. Barefoot

DEATH BY DIET

The Relationship Between Nutrient Deficiency and Disease
By Robert R. Barefoot

Published By:
Pan American International Nutrition Ltd, Publishing
Post Office Box 21389
Wickenburg, AZ 85358

All rights reserved. This publication is protected by copyright, and permission must be obtained fron the publisher prior to any prohibited reproduction, storage in a retrieval system, or transmission in any form or by any means, electronic, mechanical, photocopying, recording, or likewise. For information regarding permissions, write to:

Pan American International Nutrition Ltd, Publishing
Post Office Box 21389
Wickenburg, AZ 85358

Copyright © 2008 by Robert R. Barefoot, 1st Printing 1996, 2nd Revised Printing 1997, 3rd Revised Printing 1999, 4th Revised Printing January 2002, 5th Printing October 2002, 6th Revised Printing July 2008. Printed in the United States Of America.

Library of Congress Cataloging in Publication Data

Barefoot, Robert R.
Death By Diet, The Relationship Between Nutrient Deficiency and Disease, by Robert R. Barefoot — 5th Edition
Bibliography
Includes subjects:
1. History of Science and Medicine
2. The Food and Drug Administration
3. The Vitamin and Mineral Supplement Arguments
4. The Body's Fluids and Nutrients
5. The Human Cell
6. The Cholesterol Argument
7. The Calcium Factor in Health
8. Can Calcium Cure Cancer
9. Non Food Earth Nutrients
10. Kombucha Nutrients
11. The Carl J. Reich, M.D. Story
12. Constitutional Amendment to Include Freedom of Medicine

C.I.P.   96-84395
ISBN   978-0-9633703-3-4
Printed in the United States

TABLE OF CONTENTS

BOOK REVIEWS

*"As a result of reading the books **The Calcium Factor** and **Death By Diet**, I received excellent treatment and eventually cured myself of prostate cancer. I strongly endorse Mr. Barefoot as one of the top people in his area having excellent knowledge of nutritional therapy. I have yet to find anyone who has written such well-reasoned and scientifically based material."* David G McLean, Chairman of the Board, Canadian National Railways.

*"In October 1996 I was diagnosed with prostate cancer. The diagnosis was confirmed by biopsy. In October of that year I started following Robert Barefoot's calcium regime. In July 1997 I had another prostate biopsy in which no evidence of malignancy was found. The regime outlined in the books **The Calcium Factor** and **Death By Diet** improves the immune system to where the body can heal itself, without intrusive measures like surgery, chemotherapy or radiation."* S. Ross Johnson, Retired President of Prudential Insurance Company of America.

"I am a physician, with extensive credentials and honors that reach the White House and Heads of States in other countries. Mr. Robert Barefoot has worked over the past 20 years with many medical doctors The information has been culminated in two books, 'The Calcium Factor' and 'Death by Diet' which have been used technically as Bibles of Nutrition. Mr. Barefoot is an amazing and extraordinary man who is on a 'Great Mission' for all mankind. I thank God for Robert Barefoot." Liska M. Cooper, M.D.

*"Robert Barefoot's knowledge of calcium and its alkalizing properties has been hungrily received by 100,000's of people throughout the world who are crying out to regain their lost health and vitality. Through his books **The Calcium Factor** and **Death By Diet** he has reached out to the common man in a language he can understand."* Jill M. Wood, President Idaho Breast Implant Information Group.

INTERNET REVIEWS
(amazon.com)

"The most important health book I have ever read."
(philratte @ webtv.net, Minneapolis, Minnesota, May 19, 1999).
"This book proves how important it is to have the body fluids slightly alkaline and tells you how to test yourself so you maintain proper balance. It also proves that calcium is the most important nutrient after oxygen and water. Over 200 diseases, cancer, heart disease, diabetes, etc., are linked to Ionic Calcium Deficiency. Calcium deficiency is the universal property of all cancer cells. Moreover, the production of mutation receptors cannot occur with the pH of the cell at the healthy, calcium buffered pH of 7.4.

"A Must Reading for those who lack calcium in their diet."
(oli@omninfotech.com, May 30, 1999).
"I was born a 'Jelly Baby' and did not walk until I was four years old. All through the years I have searched for the source of Calcium that works for my body. Mr. Barefoot certainly opened my eyes on the simple reality of a healthy body. He educated me on the most beneficial kind of calcium and how it is effectively absorbed in the body. Interestingly, he further introduced me to a simple technique in finding out the level of my health. I cannot tolerate lactose and the kind of Calcium he described in his book, which I am now using, is 'Heaven Sent.' Thank you!"

"Turned My Life Around." (Russell Vandorn, russell@newonthe net.com, California, October 12, 1999).
*"I have been taking supplements for 20 years and engaged in athletic activities and working out. All was fine until a few years ago my body took a dive for no apparent reason. I tried lots of solutions with some help. Thirty days ago I read the book **The Calcium Factor** and then as instructed, acquired supplements. Like magic, the brown spots faded, my yellowing skin vanished, I lost excess weight, I regained new strength, my hair stopped falling out in the shower, I no longer get winded during exercise, and my eyesight is*

improving. I am positively amazed at what a dramatic effect the right calcium formulation has had on me. I really feel as if I'm growing younger. My friends notice it too. If you do not at least read this book, which explains everything in qualifiable scientific detail, at least take supplements, the new age antidote to aging.

"Spellbinding Information." (Nanjean, California, Dec. 13, 1999). *"I could not put this book down. In* **The Calcium Factor***, Robert Barefoot explains everything so clearly and everyone can understand this very important information. I want to scream 'WHY don't more doctors know this or pass this on!' The research was done over 60 years ago and the medical profession continues to only burn, cut or poison (radiation, surgery, chemotherapy/drugs) the symptoms of disease like it was designed to do. As the back cover of the book states, 'cancer cells cannot exist in an alkaline environment,' so if we put the body back into an alkaline state as it was when we were born, the cancer cells simply die off. Pass this book on to EVERYONE you know."*

"The greatest preventive medicine book and real eye opener!" (betcruse@webtv.net, Bay City Oregon, November 9, 1999). *I cannot extol this book enough! I have learned more in this little 138 page paperback called* **Death By Diet** *than I have in ALL the books, pamphlets, brochures, etc. that I have ever read. The knowledge, info and formulas for taking charge and gaining control of your own body's health and preventing disease is priceless! Makes complete sense. Robert Barefoot does an excellent job in explaining the technical parts of this book (remember, he is a chemist). My next book will be* **The Calcium Factor** *(same author).*

"A very important, excellent book on health." (philratte@webtv.net, Minneapolis, Minnesota, May 19, 1999). *"When I first read this book,* **Death by Diet***, I was a little skeptical about some of the ideas presented. But now that I have used some of these ideas myself, I am most impressed with their importance for my health. I have also read his new book,* **The Calcium Factor***, and it is even better. I love these books."*

ENDORSEMENTS

"Mr. Barefoot is one of the nation's top nutritional therapists, a chemist, scientist in the fields of biochemistry, hydrocarbon extraction and metal extraction from ores, inventor and holder of numerous patents, public speaker, writer, and outstanding business entrepreneur, a man of great integrity, enthusiasm, determination, loyalty, and tireless energy, coupled with a great personality. Mr. Barefoot has achieved wide acclaim in recent years for his biochemistry research into the interrelationship between disease and malnutrition, espousing that degenerative diseases are caused by mineral and vitamin deficiencies," Howard W. Pollock, Congressman (Alaska) Retired, Past President Safari Club International, Ducks Unlimited, and The National Rifle Association.

"I have been a practicing physician for the past 25 years. I am a fellow of the American College of OB-GYN and a diplomat of the American Board of OB-GYN. Mr. Barefoot has helped me immensely to understand the complex chemistry of how calcium and other minerals contribute to overall health and preventive medicine. I personally know of many individuals who are much healthier today because of Mr. Barefoot's nutritional advice, including myself." Wayne Weber M.D., Family Planning Associates Medical Group Inc., Los Angeles, California.

"I am a heart surgeon at Westchester Medical Center in Valhalla, New York, one of the largest open-heart surgery centers in the United States. I have had a special interest in nutrition over the past 30 years and have lectured on this subject throughout the United States, particularly its relationship to heart disease and other degenerative diseases. It is in this capacity that I have come to know and respect Robert Barefoot. He is an internationally known chemist with numerous international patents. His use of biochemistry in the field of hydrocarbon extraction and the field of

metal extraction of ores led him to pursue a different line of research over the past two decades, elucidating the intimate relationship between nutrition and disease," Richard W. Pooley, Professor of Surgery, New York Medical College, New York.

"I am a physician, President and Executive Medical Director of Health Insight, S.B.S. and Health Advocate Inc., in the State of Michigan. I have extensive credentials and honors that reach the White House and Heads of States in other countries. Mr. Robert Barefoot is a remarkable gentleman and a scholar who works endlessly to complete his mission to cure America. He has worked over the past 20 years with many medical doctors and scientists across the United States and in other countries doing Ortho-molecular Research on various diseases. The information has been culminated in two books, 'The Calcium Factor' and 'Death by Diet' which have been used technically as Bibles of Nutrition. Many people I know have thanked Mr. Barefoot for both saving their lives and returning them to good health. Mr. Barefoot is an amazing and extraordinary man who is on a 'Great Mission' for all mankind. I thank God for Robert Barefoot," Liska M. Cooper, M.D., Detroit, Michigan.

"I am a physician practicing at the Molecular/Biological level for over 25 years. I lecture extensively in the nutritional-medical field in Canada, the United States and Internationally. I have attended hundreds of lectures and seminars covering the aspects of medicine including a number of those given by Robert Barefoot whose discourses easily classify as absolutely excellent! Personal conversations with this man, a highly moral and ethical person, have served to confirm his unusual knowledge in the field of biologically applied nutrition and immunity enhancement." C.T. Taylor, M.D., L.M.C.C., P. Eng., Stony Plain, Alberta.

"I have been an attorney involved in very complex litigation involving natural supplements and their ability to treat or cure various types of illnesses, including cancer. I am well known in

Maryland as a litigator, repeatedly being named as one of the outstanding trial attorneys, specializing in complex matters of all natures and have written concerning trial techniques. Mr. Barefoot was engaged as an expert in the use of natural supplements, specifically minerals, and their effect on various forms of cancers. He is a renowned author in this field. There have been many occasions when I found him to be extraordinarily knowledgeable in this field of expertise. My professional opinion is that Mr. Barefoot's knowledge and experience with minerals and other natural substances and their application for the treatment of illnesses is unique. In fact, I am not aware of any other individual who possesses the knowledge and expertise in this very important and expanding field as Mr. Barefoot," David Freishtat, Attorney, Freishtat & Sandler, Baltimore, Maryland.

*"Mr. Barefoot has been, and continues to be, an advocate for health and natural healing through nutrition and knowledge. He has championed the cause of well over 440,000 American women and children who have been exposed to the toxic effects of silicone implanted devices. Mr. Barefoot, one of the rare silica chemists in the world, has delivered a message of hope to these suffering individuals, who didn't have any hope before, but are now arming themselves with the books **"The Calcium Factor"** and **"Death By Diet"** and are spreading the word. The name Barefoot has become a household word. In the past three years, he has traveled to countless meetings and medical conferences throughout the country without charging for his services. Robert Barefoot is a humanitarian and his efforts to educate through his books, informational tapes, lectures and vast media appearances has set a standard of excellence that is well above the norm. His work with hundreds of scientists and medical doctors, researching diet, has elevated him to one of the top speakers on nutrition in the nation,"* Jill M. Wood, President Idaho Breast Implant Information Group, Boise Idaho.

"I recently retired as President and CEO of Bioflora International Inc., a manufacturer of nutritional supplements, liquid mineral extracts, and liquid organic plant foods. I oversaw the

*formulation and production what is considered the world's best selling mineral supplement. I was originally introduced to and very impressed by the work of Robert Barefoot, specifically **The Calcium Factor** in 1996 but was not afforded the pleasure of a personal introduction until 1998. By that time he had developed a reputation and a title, "The King of Calcium,"* G. Scott Miller, Past President & CEO, Bioflora, Phoenix, Arizona.

"I graduated from Harvard University in 1942 (BSc Chemistry) and worked as a Research Director and in corporate management, Franklin Electronics Inc., and have been awarded two patents. Mr. Barefoot has been highly influential in my survival of prostate cancer, with which I was diagnosed in the fall of 1991. Because of his detailed knowledge of biochemistry, he has much more penetrating knowledge of the relationship between disease and nutrition, a knowledge not available to many trained dieticians because of their lack of biochemical background. With his expertise, he has aided me in not only arresting the progression of my disease, cancer, through diet and nutrition, but also reversing it. Mr. Barefoot is, simply put, an extraordinary individual," Philip Sharples, President Sharples Industries Inc., Tubac, Arizona.

"I have known Bob Barefoot for three years during which time he has provided my spouse with critical information. As a result of this relationship, I was able to introduce dozens of people to Mr. Barefoot's idea relative to critical illness and nutrition. The results achieved have been remarkable. It is my personal opinion that Mr. Barefoot is the absolute top of his field, nutritional therapy," W. Grant Fairley, The Fairley Erker Group, Edmonton, Canada.

"I am a chemist and have been involved in product development, specifically nutritional supplements. I have written numerous articles and lectured throughout the United States on these products and the benefits of utilizing alternative medicine and alternative medical products within the U.S. healthcare regimen. Over the past three years I have traveled and lectured with Mr. Barefoot on numerous

occasions all over the United States. He is recognized as a world-class expert on calcium and its nutritional benefits for the human body. Mr. Barefoot blends his prestige and uncanny ability to talk to the average person in a way that allows complicated scientific subjects to be completely understandable and accepted. I have seen Mr. Barefoot's information help a lot of people," Alex Nobles, Executive Vice President, Benchmark USA Inc., Salt Lake.

"I have been associated with Mr. Barefoot since 1993. His nutrition therapy is the result of twenty years of research into noninvasive treatment of generic diseases. In Canada we now have six M.D.s practicing his protocols. I understand that numerous Russian M.D.s in Moscow are also practicing his protocols. This number will increase exponentially as the testimonial success of hundreds of afflicted people becomes known. Mr. Barefoot's biochemistry and science brings credence to his recommended dietary and lifestyle protocols. He must be considered at the top of his field," Peter Epp. P. Eng., President Albritco Development Corporation, Calgary, Canada.

"I am the General Manager of an audio cassette tape manufacturer. Previously, I was the Vice President of an engineering consulting company specializing in nuclear technology analysis under contract to the U.S. government. With a BS degree in Electrical Engineering, graduate schoolwork at UCLA and over 10 years of research at McDonnell Douglas, my technical and scientific tools are extensive. I currently specialize in the audio production of technical information specializing in nutrition and health. It is in this regard that I have come to know the reputation and work of Robert Barefoot. Our company actively seeks men and women with scientific and medical backgrounds in order to develop substantive resource material for our client base. Robert Barefoot's lectures, books and tapes support his position as a leading spokesperson for the benefits of nutrition for good health," Al Vendetti, General Manager, Exxel Audio Productions, Oceanside, California.

"I am the founder of a company that specializes in both mining and the export of health and nutritional products overseas. Mr. Barefoot has tremendous knowledge of biochemistry and his expertise in the field of calcium research has earned him recognition worldwide for both his lecturing and his research. He has authored several books, which my company exports overseas as nutritional standards for people involved in the nutrition industry. He has also researched and developed calcium supplements, which are being exported to several countries abroad. His research of the relationship between disease and nutrition is gaining recognition worldwide and if properly implemented, could substantially reduce the devastating effects of degenerative diseases caused by mineral and vitamin deficiency," Brett R. Davies, President, Davies International, Denver, Colorado.

"I am well-known in the area of nutrition. I am certified by the National Association of Health Care Professionals as a Health Care Councilor and have lectured extensively in the United States, Canada, Russia and the Ukraine. Mr. Barefoot is considered one of the most knowledgeable people in the world on effects of calcium on health," Robert G. Bremner, Mechanicsville, Virginia.

"Mr. Barefoot is a man in pursuit of "Excellence" in all his endeavors. He has received wide recognition for his research in the biochemistry field, dealing with malnutrition. I have the distinct privilege and pleasure of having known Mr. Barefoot for several years," Jerry R. Gallion, International Financier, Vaulx Milieu, France.

"I am a retired university professor, Ph.D., known in the field of Pharmaceutical Chemistry, having written and lectured extensively over a forty-year period, publishing numerous scientific articles. Based on Mr. Barefoot's education, and background in chemistry and nutrition, along with his published books and lecturing, it is my professional opinion that Mr. Barefoot is near the top of his field," Jerry Rollins, PhD, Austin, Texas.

FOREWORD

"If the doctors of today do not become the nutritionists of tomorrow, then the nutritionists of today will become the doctors of tomorrow."

--- Rockefeller Institute of Medical Research

DEATH BY DIET was written by popular request as a sequel to, and includes many excerpts from, the book **THE CALCIUM FACTOR**, by Bob Barefoot and Carl J. Reich, M.D., in which the authors gave a detailed technical defense to the concept that most degenerative diseases are caused by mineral and vitamin deficiency. In their book they tie scientific evidence provided by some of the world's most renowned scientists together into one cohesive scientific argument that demonstrates that *nutritional deficiency not only is the cause of disease, but that by correcting the deficiency, disease can not only be prevented, but also cured.* This practice of preventive medicine is not very popular among the leaders of the medical establishment, as the book shows how medical pioneers who dare to practice preventive medicine are slowly ostracized and criticized prior to the removal of their license to practice medicine. The technical arguments in this book are the collection of accepted scientific facts, and are presented in a manner to rebut biased criticism. This makes some of the chapters difficult reading for the layperson, many of whom have requested a follow-up book that could be read easily by the general public.

DEATH BY DIET was written to include many of the scientific arguments in a language that the reader could understand and appreciate, supporting preventive medicine through nutritional management. Those wishing more technical substance can purchase the book, **THE CALCIUM FACTOR**, at:

866-723-2551

DEATH BY DIET was written for three main reasons: **first**, to inform the American public that *mineral and vitamin deficiency is the main cause of degenerative disease,* **second**, to explain to the public that *a medical freedom amendment to the Constitution will be necessary to change the current restrictive, disease-dependent system,* and **third**, to suggest to the politicians that *the promotion of preventive medicine could lead to the cure for many of America's current economic woes and could result in massive savings in health care expenditures* (the drug industry raked in over $700 billion in 1994, and over $1,300 billion in 1996), *tens of billions of dollars every year* (for example, in 1994, heart disease alone cost Americans an estimated $128 billion that included charges for physicians, nursing, hospital, nursing home services along with medication and the value of time lost from work), which *would dramatically **reduce the deficit** while making the voters both happy and healthy.*

Deficiencies of critical minerals, such as calcium and magnesium, that are combined with a deficiency of vitamin D, cause the body fluids, which are normally mildly alkaline, to become acidic. It is this "*acidosis*" that is the cause of heart disease, cancer, arthritis, osteoporosis and numerous other degenerative diseases. Although the importance of minerals and vitamins is becoming more and more recognized, the missing ingredient, vitamin D, is almost never recommended in amounts that will ensure that the body absorbs them. The book provides simple technical explanations in terms easily understood, identifying what causes degenerative diseases, with support from world-renowned scientists, as well as descriptions of biochemical mechanisms. The book will show that *the current **Recommended Daily Allowances** (RDAs) of vitamins and minerals are **ridiculously low***, encouraging disease, and are in contradiction to many exhaustive and massive scientific studies. The book will show that the medical regulatory system, which has a dismal track record and thrives on the economics of disease, is allowed to systematically persecute, with cries of "*quackery*" and "*charlatan*," those who seek to research and promote preventive medicine. Because of the lack of medical freedom in America, knowledgeable doctors are fearful of losing their licenses if they break from the system and practice preventive medicine. Finally, the book will explain that with a change in lifestyle and only pennies' worth of food supplements, a means of both preventing and curing degenerative disease exists which can be monitored for just one penny per day.

Changing the system of managed medicine that has been in place for hundreds of years is a formidable task, equivalent to moving a mountain. There are those that would like to see the system changed, but advocate a program of slowly chipping away at the mountain in a manner that will not disturb its current inhabitants. There are many more, however, that would like to see it done in their lifetimes, and thereby realize that to accomplish their goal, some "*establishment-awakening*" explosives will be necessary.

Unfortunately, there is no way to change the system that perpetuates the maintenance of disease by diet without attacking those who have a vested economic interest in defending the system. These establishment regulators mean well and were not responsible for the system into which they were born. An examination of both medical and scientific history will show that it was the system in which they governed that allowed the establishment to resist most of the advances of science that all human societies now believe to be basic truths of life. This resistance to change was done while vilifying and demeaning some of the many famous men in history, most of whom are now referred to as the fathers of science. These world-renowned men made major scientific contributions that can lead to the understanding and prevention of disease.

One such famous man was two-time winner of the Nobel Prize in Medicine, 1931 and 1944, Otto Warburg. He proved that anaerobism, the lack of oxygen, was the cause of cancer, and in 1966 ,when he was the Director of Max Planck Institute for Cell Physiology, Berlin, he presented a paper to the Nobel Laureates at Lindau, Germany entitled *"The Prime Cause and Prevention of Cancer."* Warburg stated, **"There is no disease whose prime cause is better known,"** so that today ignorance is no longer an excuse that one cannot do more about prevention of cancer. But how long prevention will be avoided depends on how long the prophets of agnosticism (the belief that nothing is known) will succeed in inhibiting the application of scientific knowledge in the field of cancer. **In the meantime millions of men and women must die of cancer unnecessarily."** (Note: in 1966 cancer struck 23% of Americans, whereas today it strikes 39% of Americans). **"How many more must needlessly die?"** (Otto Warburg)

It is hoped that this book will help both the doctors and the public to better understand disease so that society can change the present disease care system into a real health care system by practicing preventive medicine, thereby allowing the human race to change the current trend of *death by diet.*

PREFACE

Although **DEATH BY DIET** outlines the shameful track record of the medical establishment system, it is not intended to be critical or judgmental of the medical doctors themselves, most of whom either believe in, or would like to learn more about, the practice of preventive medicine, but are threatened with having their licenses revoked if they do so. The examples given in **DEATH BY DIET** of the medical and scientific communities are *historical facts*, and are not meant to demean either profession. The author has many close friends in, and the greatest respect for, both professions. *All criticisms* are directed at the few in the *upper echelon of the governing bureaucratic establishments,* who rigidly regulate the innovation of doctors and scientists while vigorously protecting their own prestigious status quo empires. Unfortunately, criticism of these elite and most respected men is often met with the blind and defensive cry of *"blasphemy,"* thereby providing encouragement for the system to perpetuate its mistakes at the cost of human lives and suffering. This may sound like an exaggeration, but history teaches us that it is not. The medical authorities prevented the doctors throughout the world from washing their hands after autopsies and surgeries *for decades after scientific evidence was presented* that showed that by not washing his hands, the physician

xviii

could cause the death of his patient. Large numbers of American citizens suffered and were killed by this policy while the fear of blasphemy protected the medical establishment from criticism. Ironically, blasphemy is, *"the disrespect for persons or things regarded as **sacred**."* This implies that such men are **holy** and therefore incapable of making mistakes. Even **they** know that this is not true. It is hoped that by pointing out some of their mistakes, both they and the reader will be alerted to the fact that history may be once again repeating itself in a tragic fashion.

Only about one in three doctors in America belong to the American Medical Association (the AMA). Why? I have been told by some that it is because of its dismal record. The public is also expressing its concern, as over 60 percent of Americans are currently seeking alternative medicine, according to one current CBS documentary on the state of medicine in America. One of the AMA's most important mandates is to protect the public. But from whom? **"Charlatans and quacks"** is the answer, according to their historical performance. The only problem with this noble mandate is that those who are empowered to make the decision are not only judge and jury, but also very biased and usually ignorant of certain medical facts. If new, non-orthodox and inexpensive medical procedures are introduced, these jurors are challenged in two ways: First, their historical adherence to status quo medicine will put their medical expertise into question with the general public, and second, their bountiful financial empires will be threatened. The irony behind this is that it is not their fault. They were born into the system that did not enshrine freedom of medicine in their Constitution. The result has been the erosion of medical management into a **guilty-until-proven-innocent** stance, which, due to the enormous financial burden necessary to provide proof, does not allow the individual medical pioneer to defend his position. If the medical authorities are really trying to unbiasedly protect the public, then they should stop chasing medical charlatans and unleash their massive financial *power to protect the public from poor health and disease* by researching what the medical entrepreneurs have to offer. The medical pioneer should be innocent until proven guilty, and the onus should be on the AMA to prove him either right or wrong, for by doing so, it would be serving the public's best interest.

Many doctors and nutritionists contend that the AMA's claim that it is looking after the *"health care"* of America is both incorrect and misleading. In reality, they are looking after the *"disease care"* of America. Unfortunately, caring for disease is very profitable, while preventing disease is not. For every dollar spent on health, more than ten is spent on disease, proving once again that an ounce of prevention is worth a pound of cure. Thus, *real health care implies the endorsement of preventive medicine*, which must include the nutritional therapy that the AMA is currently impeding.

How did America create this disease-care society? Well, it happened because, 220 years ago, Americans lost their rights to one of life's basic freedoms: *the freedom of medicine*—the freedom for each American citizen *to choose* and *to practice* the form of medicine that the citizen deems most beneficial to his personal health. Freedom of medicine was tragically left out of the American Constitution. In 1776, Dr. Benjamin Rush, America's first Surgeon General and the only American doctor to sign the Declaration of Independence, was responsible for the inclusion of *freedom of religion* and also tried strenuously—but failed—to have *"medical freedom"* enshrined in the Constitution. He feared that, *"the time will come when medicine will organize into an undercover dictatorship*." He estimated it would happen within 60 years, and his fears were well founded, as in 1839 the AMA was founded and immediately began to ostracize the then-popular, and what was referred to as the *"enemy"*—homeopathic doctors from its medical ranks. Doctors were even disbarred from hospitals where homeopaths practiced. Even before the formation of the AMA, orthodox doctors had seized powerful positions of prestige. Unfortunately, George Washington was one of their early victims. Washington was bled to death by the then-orthodox medical practice of *blood letting*. This early AMA medical practice of *shunning the competition* would be strictly illegal today — in every field except medicine. Any doctor today getting caught following the father of medicine, Hippocrates' examples of preventive medicine and of letting the patients decide, is currently in danger of having his license revoked. This is done in the name of public protection. Tragically, the real protection is for the staggeringly high profits of the drug companies.

It is therefore obvious that the only corrective prescription to cure the ills of modern medicine would be an amendment to the American Constitution, enshrining *medical freedom and* thereby allowing every citizen the right to choose and the right to practice the form of medicine that the citizen deems most beneficial to his personal health. This would, in effect, be setting free the citizen with the *right to choose* and the physician with the *right to practice* any and all forms of medicine.

ABOUT THE AUTHOR

In 1963, when Bob Barefoot was 19-years-old, he read an article that was to change his outlook on life. The article by a McGill University scientist was about research relating to calcium depletion of the bones, and how this process paralleled aging. The article suggested that if the process could be slowed down chemically, so too would the process of aging, thereby suggesting that the secrets of calcium depletion could lead to the *fountain of youth*.

Mr. Barefoot became a chemist specializing in mineral diageneses, which is the process by which minerals are constantly changing from one form to another; Mr. Barefoot researched and published scientific articles on the subject. He later began researching metal extraction in the mining industry, for which he obtained a number of international patents. He also researched enhanced hydrocarbon extraction in the petroleum industry. All the time he was doing this chemical research, he was aggressively amassing all the technical publications he could find concerning biochemical calcium. Ironically, he found that if he was to be successful in the mining and petroleum industries, an advanced understanding of the chemistry of calcium was necessary, as calcium is a major and active constituent in geology. Mr. Barefoot experimented with altering and creating compounds and minerals, such as calcium phosphate (apatite), which is also the major constituent of bones. He found that to accomplish this within the hydrocarbon reservoir, chemically buffered solutions, much like the ones in the human body, had to be developed. Thus, over the years, Mr. Barefoot amassed a great deal of advanced chemical knowledge and was up-to-date with the leaders in the scientific community when he fortuitously, or *by fate*, met Dr. Carl J. Reich.

Dr. Reich was known as a medical maverick who had pioneered in mineral deficiency-related diseases for over thirty years. By changing the lifestyles of his patients and giving them mineral and vitamin supplements, he was able to turn their lives around. As word of his successes grew, his practice flourished. He tried to share the fruits of his research with his medical peers. However, they reacted in typical historical fashion, and shunned him as if he had the plague and crowned him with the title *"quack."* He continued to develop clinical procedures and to successfully treat thousands of grateful patients who had received no benefit from orthodox medicine, until finally, he had gone too far. While his patients all loved him, his medical peers began to dutifully complain to the medical licensing authorities, and so, after thirty-two years of practice, his license was suspended. Undaunted, he continued to research and seek out those with knowledge about minerals and the human body.

Barefoot was absolutely astounded by the knowledge and experience amassed by Dr. Reich, especially the valuable information that was attained from the doctor-only medical libraries. He set out to search for publications that supported the views of Dr. Reich and found that scientific and medical literature abounded with such information. Even more astounding was the fact that

Dr. Reich's personal files abounded with proof that he had cured cancer using nutritional therapy. Medical records of his patients showed that terminal cancer patients had come to him in a last ditch effort to save their lives. Dr. Reich treated them with nutritional therapy, especially vitamin D and calcium supplements, and when they finally died several years later, autopsies showed that they died of natural causes, and *did not have cancer.* Furthermore, in the early sixties, Dr. Reich had presented his thesis to the Max Plank Institute in Berlin that the cancer cell was not absolutely anoxic, but only functionally anoxic due to calcium deficiency, and therefore could not utilize the oxygen in its environment. This intrigued two-time Nobel Prize winner, Otto Warburg agreed to collaborate with Dr. Reich on his research. Unfortunately, Dr. Warburg died before the work could be completed. Carl then spent the next 20 years searching for a chemist to assist him. Then he met Barefoot and both men eagerly agreed to collaborate and share their experiences and discoveries by writing a book that compiled the scientific evidence in a manner that medical authorities could not refute without refuting the work of many world-renowned scientists. The result was the 1992 publication of **THE CALCIUM FACTOR**.

The book proved to spark much technical interest and was well received by those who read it, receiving many silent accolades from doctors who claimed that they feared being involved in public endorsement of the book. Only one doctor to date has been negative. He claimed to represent the authorities and wanted to know if Mr. Barefoot was not, *"afraid of going to jail for practicing medicine without a license."* Mr. Barefoot responded that if dispensing technical information to the public on the practice of preventive medicine is considered to be practicing medicine, then *why was he himself not practicing medicine*, as he was supposed to be the doctor? He replied, *"They said that you would have all of the answers,"* as he slammed the phone down. This enjoyable experience has been overshadowed by even more enjoyable comments from those in the scientific community who agreed that, *"You are definitely on the right track."* However, the general public responded that they had difficulty understanding the book, even though they could see from the massive scientific references that Mr. Barefoot must be correct. It is for these people that **DEATH BY DIET** was written.

ACKNOWLEDGMENT

The author is grateful and wishes to acknowledge his appreciation for the contribution and efforts of his best friends: John and Isabel Baker of Big Valley, Alberta; Bruce and Carole Downey of Wickenburg, Arizona; Dr. Carl Reich and Peter Epp of Calgary, Canada; Ed Will of Congress, Arizona; and the author's dear wife Karen, who resides with the author in Wickenburg, Arizona.

NOTATION

This publication is intended to direct the attention of both the physician and the patient to the torrent of scientific research being carried out on the significance of nutrition in preventive medicine. It is not the intention of the author to provide an alternative to the orthodox physician-patient relationship. It is the objective of the author *to expand the dimensions of orthodox medicine itself*, and help speed it towards the medical practices of the twenty-first century where diet and lifestyle will play a dominant role in preventive medicine (Carl J. Reich, M.D., Father of Preventive Medicine).

CHAPTER ONE

IN THE BEGINNING

It is said that one of the most important reasons for learning history is because *history repeats itself,* and therefore, *to know history is to know the future.* The reason for this phenomenon is that humans are both creatures of habit and of predictable emotions that preside over logic. Thus, we find that the trends in medical history both follow and parallel the trends in scientific history where many a genius has been destroyed by people of lesser talent defending the status quo. Therefore, before judging medical innovators, it is necessary to put them in historical perspective so their views are not clouded by the biased authoritarian establishment, whose track record leaves a lot to be desired.

"Innovation is a two-fold threat to the scientific hierarchy. First, it threatens their oracle authority. Secondly, it evokes the deeper fear that their whole laboriously constructed authoritarian edifice may collapse." (Arthur Koestler, *The Age of Velikovsky*).

"Great spirits have always encountered violent opposition from mediocre minds." (Albert Einstein).

1

About 2,500 years ago, a man named Hippocrates wrote a detailed manual for medicine, outlining the duties, obligations and responsibilities of being a doctor. It is ironic that every doctor today swears to the Hippocratic Oath, and then proceeds to practice medicine that does not include Hippocrates' basic teachings on preventive medicine:

*"All food is medicine, and the best food is the best medicine. Sunshine and fresh air must be considered as good food. Please don't worry, as worrying is not considered to be a good food, and besides, medical science has made marvelous advances over the past hundreds of years, and we are now at the point where we can do a great deal to help **cure diseases such as cancer.**"* (*Hippocrates*, father of medicine).

Wow! A 2,500 year old cure for cancer! And he did it by prescribing large doses of garlic and onions. It was a good thing that Dr. Hippocrates was prescribing such things before the American Medical Association (AMA) was formed, or he most assuredly would have become a target of medical shunning and had his license to practice medicine suspended for practicing **"medical quackery**." Today, the medical authorities would demand that Dr. Hippocrates prove scientifically with massive and expensive scientific and public testing, that his claims were valid. In Hippocrates' day, he only had to prove it to his patients. Since no individual man would have the resources to do this (probably requiring tens of millions of dollars), the medical authorities, claiming that they are **protecting the public**, win by default, while the public loses the right to pursue preventive medicine. It is ironic because the AMA does have the resources to prove whether the claim is valid, but refuses, putting the onus on the claimant. Thus nothing is or can be done, and the American public is protected from Hippocrates' garlic and onions.

2

Tragically, there is a history of scientific evidence that garlic and onions may indeed act as a retardant in the prevention of cancer. The scientific community recently sent a team of scientists to China to study the phenomenon that, in locations where millions of Chinese eat large amounts of garlic and onions, stomach cancer virtually does not exist. This is especially stunning as cancer strikes one out of every three people in the West. Scientists have been able to extract certain *sulfur components* from both garlic and onions, which they found to be *extremely powerful antibiotics* and probably *anti-carcinogenic*. In line with the standard medical thinking of the day, they are currently attempting to economically extract the active components so that the drug companies can produce another expensive new white powder for consumption by the American public. Meanwhile, Hippocrates is probably rolling in his grave shouting, *"Why don't you just let them eat the damned garlic and onions?"*

The calamity is compounded by the fact that there is also an abundant and readily available history of scientific evidence, demonstrating that garlic and onions also have proven properties beneficial to health. In a recent *Scientific American* publication, *The Chemistry of Garlic and Onions*, Eric Block, University of Saint Louis, describes how certain extracts of both garlic and onions have proven to be *antibacterial, antifungal, and antithrombotic* (keeps blood from clotting, which is very important in certain surgical procedures, such as transplanting body organs). Block skillfully tracks history, from Hippocrates to the Egyptian pharaohs, who were entombed with garlic and onions, to the black plague of the middle ages, where those handling the millions of diseased and contagious bodies drank a daily concoction of garlic and spirits, which resulted in none of them dying; to Louis Pasteur, who, in 1858, reported that garlic is antibacterial; to Chester J. Cavallito, who, in 1944, established that an oil extracted from garlic (later identified as diallyl disulfide oxide) was not only antibacterial and antifungal, but was also *more potent than*

3

penicillin against B. thyosis; to Albert Schweitzer, who used garlic in Africa for treating dysentery and to prevent gangrene. The current scientific literature contains a litany of other evidence on the benefits of garlic and onions. Despite all this overwhelming evidence, the current medical authorities can be heard issuing their standard prewritten script, "*Very interesting, but we do not think that there is enough scientific evidence either to show what the long-term effects will be on human health, or to merit our pursuing the matter at this time.*"

Dr. Sidney Belman, professor of Environmental Medicine at New York University Medical Center, found that applying garlic oil to mice that had been exposed to a cancer-causing chemical prevented them from developing skin tumors. He reported his findings in 1983 in the journal *Carcinogenesis*. Subsequent studies of large populations of people support such animal studies. In the *Journal of the National Cancer Institute* (1989) for example, U.S. and Chinese scientists reported on a study of residents of a particular region of China. They found that the more people ate garlic and onions, the less likely they were to develop stomach cancer—the most common cause of death among cancer patients on a global scale. Inspired by Bellman's work, Dr. Michael Wargovich at the University of Texas M.D. Anderson Cancer Center in Houston has been studying a particular garlic component as an inhibitor of digestive-tract tumors. When his colleagues learned that Wargovich was involved in garlic research, he said, "The people who were in chemotherapy, they sort of rolled their eyes."

Despite all this overwhelming evidence, the current medical authorities can be seen "rolling their eyes" and can be heard issuing their standard pre-written script, *"Very interesting, but we do not think that there is enough scientific evidence either to show what the long-term effects will be on human health, or to merit our pursuing the matter at this time."*

4

Another Hippocratic argument that must be addressed is the statement that *"sunshine must be considered as **good food**"* and therefore is *"**good medicine**."* The medical authorities of today have everyone convinced that sunshine *causes* skin cancer, and is therefore bad for you. Nothing could be further from the truth. In later chapters it will be explained how sunshine not only does not cause cancer, but how sunshine actually *prevents* cancer. The oversimplification in current medical thinking has done a disservice to the teachings of Hippocrates, which science has proven correct. Besides, the implication that the sun causes cancer implies that God did not know what he was doing to the health of humans when He created the sun.

One of the sad realities of ignoring history is that almost every American is ignorant of the fact that medical freedom was tragically left out of the American Constitution. In 1776, Dr. Benjamin Rush, Surgeon General and the only American doctor to sign the Declaration of Independence, tried strenuously, but failed, to have *"medical freedom"* enshrined in the Constitution. He feared that, "the time will come when medicine will organize into an *undercover dictatorship*." He estimated it would happen within 60 years, and his fears were well founded, as in 1839 the AMA was founded and immediately began to ostracize the then popular— and what was referred to as the *enemy*—homeopathic doctors from its medical ranks. Doctors were even disbarred from hospitals where homeopaths practiced. Even before the formation of the AMA, orthodox doctors had seized powerful positions of prestige, and, unfortunately, George Washington was one of their early victims – bled to death by the then orthodox practice of *blood letting*. This early AMA medical practice of *shunning the competition* would be strictly illegal today – in every field except medicine. Any doctor today getting caught following Hippocrates' examples of preventive medicine and letting the patients decide is in danger of having his license revoked. This is done in the name of public protection. Tragically, the real

5

protection is for the staggeringly high profits of the drug companies. It is therefore obvious that the only corrective prescription to cure the ills of modern medicine would be an *amendment to the American Constitution, enshrining medical freedom*, thereby allowing both doctors and patients the right to practice and to preach preventive medicine:

"Each and every American citizen has the right to choose and to practice the form of medicine that the citizen deems most beneficial to personal health, without economic, physical, political, or verbal interference or abuse. And any institution or governmental agency assigned to protect the state of the individual's health should be empowered only to make recommendations that do not infringe or prevent the individual's right to choose and to practice any form of medicine."

CHAPTER TWO

SCIENCE AND MEDICINE IN THE NINETEENTH CENTURY

In 1808, Dalton, the father of modern chemistry, proposed the *Atomic Theory*: Atoms were the basic components of all substances. Today, every child in every school is taught and believes the Atomic Theory to be a basic truth, as they use it to predict and measure chemical reactions. However, the scientific establishment in Dalton's day reacted by throwing scorn on his theory. For decades the sarcastic chorus of criticism continued to emanate from the establishment. Sixty-one years later, in 1869, Professor Williamson, President of the Chemical Society, "humored" those who accepted the theory stating that, "*For lack of a better theory, it will have to do for now.*" Even after one hundred years had elapsed, prominent scientists of the day, such as the renowned Professor Ostwald, were publicly administering scathing condemnations of Dalton's theories, while attempting to show that the theory of chemistry was independent of the theory of atoms. Even though the establishment was rigid in its negative opinion, one hundred years of debate had created many supporters of the theory. Lesser known scientists of the day, such as Albert Einstein and Max Planck, believed that the Atomic Theory was not only correct, but was natural as sunshine. Thus, the chemical establishment of the nineteenth century fought against a theory

7

that the chemical establishment of the twentieth century know to be a basic truth of life. It is most probable that the chemical establishment of the twenty-first century will find many of the theories that their twentieth century forefathers are currently suppressing to be basic truths of life, as *history almost always repeats itself*.

The nineteenth century also saw medical science experiencing similar resistance to change. One classic example, that caused the death of unknown multitudes of people all over the world, was the case of Dr. Semmelweis. In 1841, Ignas Semmelweis, a Hungarian physician, was horrified by the high death rate of women giving birth in hospitals and became obsessed with finding the cause of the disease.

At that time, mothers who had given birth at home or in carriages on the way to the hospital had a far greater chance of surviving their childbirth than if they had been delivered in a hospital. Women were terrified, as the death rate was staggering. Semmelweis noted that it was common practice for the doctors of the time to go directly from the morgue, where they had been conducting post-mortem examinations, and from anatomy classes using the bodies of deceased patients, into the maternity ward. He also noted that they attended maternity patients dressed in usual garb and without washing their hands. For these and other reasons, Dr. Semmelweis suspected that the doctors were carrying an agent on their hands that was causing the fatal disease. In 1847, when Semmelweis instituted a procedure in one hospital of scrubbing and dipping the doctors' hands in a chlorine solution before every procedure, the death rate fell almost immediately from thirty percent to *practically zero*. Seven other major hospitals followed suit with the same result.

The protective medical establishment of the day, embarrassed by something that they did not understand, reacted by blocking Dr. Semmelweis' applications for any further research funds, and proceeded to vilify, ostracize, and finally have him discharged from his prestigious positions in maternity hospitals. One wonders what would have happened if this all-male bastion regulating the doctors had but just one woman member, as their decision caused women to suffer and die for decades to come.

In America, the condemnation of Semmelweis was hailed by the newly formed AMA, who followed suit by threatening to remove the license of any doctor caught washing his hands. Their reasoning was that *doctors believing in things that **they could not see** was the same as doctors believing in spooks*, and therefore, a violation of the Hippocratic Oath that they all took. The medical authorities could not understand how something as simple as *the washing of hands* could have such a profound effect on medicine. Ironically, the same logic, that *it is just **too simple** to have any validity,* is being used today to suppress the use of foods as cures. Their tragic policy would prove to be, in effect, a death sentence for multitudes, perhaps millions, of Americans for decades to come.

Meanwhile, back in Europe, Dr. Semmelweis was so haunted by the fact that thousands of women were continuing to die, that he eventually died of insanity in 1865. What really makes this case so tragic is that, even when the medical establishment finally admitted its blunder almost a half century later, they did not recognize that they were repeating history by continuing to make similar tragic mistakes.

By the 1880s, the advent of the microscope made the microbe—which had once been invisible to the doctor's eye—very visible for doctors and the whole world to see. Louis Pastuer, father of the Germ Theory of Disease, and Joseph Lister father of the use of antiseptics, took pictures of bacteria using the microscope, and presented the pictures to the AMA stating, "Here are Dr. Semmelweis' *spooks*." Despite this fact, the medical authorities still refused to endorse Dr. Semmelweis' hand-washing procedure, stating that more evidence was required. The doctors, however, now unbridled by the accusation of *believing in spooks*, began to universally wash their hands, but only in hiding.

Despite this acceptance of Semmelweis' procedure by most of the doctors of the time, both Louis Pasteur and Joseph Lister encountered substantial difficulty having the *Germ Theory of Disease* lead to antiseptic surgery, as medical authorities refused to accept the theory. This position proved to be another death sentence for multitudes of Americans. Thus, the medical establishment of the nineteenth century fought against a theory that the medical establishment of the twentieth century knows to be a basic truth of life. Once again it is most probable that the medical establishment of the twenty-first century will find many of the theories that their twentieth century forefathers are currently suppressing to be basic truths of life, as *history almost always repeats itself.*

CHAPTER THREE

SCIENCE AND MEDICINE IN THE TWENTIETH CENTURY

Albert Einstein, my hero, who was unquestionably the most famous scientist of the twentieth century, had to withstand more efforts by the establishment attempting to disprove his *Theory of Relativity* than have ever been made to disprove any theory in the history of science. This was demonstrated by one of the establishment opponent's publications entitled, *"One Hundred Against Einstein."* Einstein remarked that, "If they were right, one would be enough." Thus, the scientific establishment of the beginning of the twentieth century fought against a theory that the scientific establishment later in the twentieth century knows to be one of the most important basic truths of life. Once again it is most probable that the scientific establishment of the twenty-first century will find many of the theories that their twentieth century forefathers are currently suppressing to be basic truths of life, as *history almost always repeats itself.*

Max Planck, a father of modern physics and the 1903 Nobel Prize winner, stated that, "An important scientific innovation rarely makes its way by gradually winning over and converting its opponents; what does happen is its opponents gradually die out and the growing generation is familiarized with the idea from the

11

beginning." What this means is that the opponents of preventive medicine by nutrition will have to die out. Let us hope for our children's sake that many have already done so. Planck's message is that, to be accepted, the children will have to be taught that Hippocrates was right when he said "*Food is medicine, and the best food is the best medicine*." Although the medical establishment would not dare to verbally offend the memory of Hippocrates, knowing better, they suggest that what he really meant was "eat your fruits and vegetables," while they get rich dispensing the expensive *unnatural white chemicals* of the drug companies.

A lso in the first half of the twentieth century, Theodore Boverie, *the true father of genetic science*, discovered almost every detail of cell division, including chromosomes, which, he concluded, transmit heredity. This idea was strenuously opposed by the protective establishment, led by Thomas Morgan. When, years later, he found that his own experiments agreed with Boverie's, he did the honorable thing by quietly ignoring his previous criticisms. Morgan then went on to describe the chromosome structure in more detail, adding specific positions called *"genes,"* for which he received the Nobel Prize in 1937. Once again the establishment's opposition to a new theory had been proven wrong, only this time one of their own banner carriers saved the day for them.

B y the middle of the twentieth century, science had progressed to the point where the scientific establishment of the day announced to the world that, "*In this atomic age, all there is to know has already been learned, and all future advancements will simply be rearrangements of current knowledge*." Wow! What arrogance! What these scientists needed was a history lesson so that they could be taught to understand the old adages, "The less we know, the more sure we are," and "The more we know, the less sure we are." One thing is for sure, those scientists lacked wisdom, and unfortunately, many of their replacements are displaying the same traits.

The beginning of the twentieth century also saw scientists starting to correlate the existence of bioelectrical systems with biological function. This brought gasps of horror from the governing establishment, as well as from traditional biologists, who—for the most part—were successful in removing the funding for such experimentation. The medical establishment was so miffed by these proposals that it was determined to block the propagation of *"such nonsense."* Even under this severe duress, electrobiochemistry was further researched and when the pioneers of electroencephalography (the recording of electrical brain impulses known as an EEG) and electrocardiographs employed the new procedures, they were labeled *"electronic quacks"* by the American Medical Association. Furthermore, the threat that *electronic quackery* could be used as a reason to suspend a doctor's license dissuaded most doctors from using the new procedures, and therefore resulted in much human suffering. The scientific establishment of the beginning of the twentieth century fought against a theory that the scientific establishment later in the twentieth century knows to be both valid and important to medicine as well as another basic truth of life. Once again, it is most probable that the scientific establishment of the twenty-first century will find many of the theories that the current medical forefathers are suppressing, to also be *basic truths of life*, as *history almost always repeats itself.*

More recently, in the latter part of the twentieth century, electrophysiologists, such as Dr. Robert Becker, a research orthopedic surgeon, found—as others before him had found—that he had to wage a battle against the *"frozen thinking of the establishment,"* who to this day continue to block advancements in this field. In his book, *The Body Electric*, which is full of exciting new concepts and easily the best book I have ever read,

Dr. Becker describes how the **negative current of injury** allows prepubescent children to regenerate chopped-off fingers and toes when the skin is not sutured over the stump, as long as the severance is below the last joint. The wound may be dressed but must be left open so that it will remain electrically negative, thereby allowing a **human limb to regrow**. Dr. Becker has actually been able to grow limbs on animals that currently have no regeneration possibilities, and he has good reason to believe that scientific research will one day lead to the capability of regenerating human limbs for everyone. Once again – and tragically – the system effectively blocks all research funds directed towards this **medically forbidden field.**

The concepts of limb regeneration are not new. In fact, the regeneration of the fingers and toes of prepubescent children is a common practice outside North America. It was discovered in the early 1970s by the English surgeon, Cynthia Illingworth, of the Sheffield Children's Hospital. She accidentally found, when a nurse forgot to suture a child's wound, that when a young child's finger is sheared off beyond the outermost crease of the outermost last joint, and the wound is **dressed but not closed** the finger will grow back perfectly within three months. By 1974, Illingworth documented the regrowth of several hundred fingertips. Other pediatric surgeons, like Dr. Michael Bleicher, of New York's Mount Sinai Hospital, have become confident of the infallibility of the process. Yet few hospitals accept this **natural replacement procedure**, allowing children to lose their fingertips, as it has not been endorsed by the medical authorities. It is hoped that – as Max Planck believed – when the children learn of the facts, and when the ruling establishment dies out, other human limbs, such as arms and legs, will be regrown, giving hope and reducing human pain and suffering. And, once again, the only way to speed up the procedure would be for the public to **endorse a constitutional amendment for freedom of medicine**.

Likewise, *acupuncture*, a safe and non-chemical method of reducing pain, is also not accepted by most Western doctors. Probably, the real reason is because *it was not invented here*, and because billions of dollars would potentially be lost annually. Western medicine refuses to examine the overwhelming evidence—including thousands of painless operations on people and animals—of the success of acupuncture, claiming to require a valid scientific explanation for the phenomenon. And guess what! The scientific explanation exists, but it has to be explained using the medically forbidden field of electrophysiology.

In his book, *The Body Electric*, Dr. Becker explains how pain is caused when the closed bioelectric circuit is broken. He shows how stimulating the body's electrical P-N junction points short circuits the severed system allowing the flow of electrons to continue to the brain, thereby fooling the brain into thinking that the circuit was never broken. The result is *no pain*. Now that acupuncture can be explained in terms that Western science understands, the medical authorities do not have to continue to complain that the people and animals who have used acupuncture *may be liars*. Even more astounding than Becker's explanation of acupuncture is the fact that his human map of the P-N junction points that were electrically identified matches the ancient Chinese map of the points to be stimulated by acupuncture. Although it is true that a pill in the stomach can cure a pain in the head, it is just as true that a needle in the head can cure a pain in the stomach. Unfortunately, the only way that Western medicine will allow human pain and suffering to be reduced is to pay billions to the drug companies This does not eliminate the thousands of deaths each year that are caused by the use of toxic chemical anesthetics. However, *acupuncture would eliminate most, if not all, of these needless deaths*. And again, the only way to speed up the use of acupuncture by Western medicine would be for the public to endorse a *constitutional amendment for freedom of medicine*.

By ignoring the fact that most biological functions are electrically controlled, the medical profession remains ignorant of the effects on the human body of low-frequency electromagnetic fields. The superimposition of these fields, emanating from most of the electronic gadgetry of our day, over the natural bioelectric fields in the human body, causes a change in the electric field, thereby altering their functions and inducing ill health. This emanating of low frequency electromagnetic fields is known as *electropollution*, and will become one of the most important topics discussed in the twenty-first century.

Any discussion of medicine in the twentieth century would be incomplete without the mention of the positive advances in medicine. The first was the discovery of the *"natural"* bacterial agent, penicillin, which is still the most effective antibiotic *"drug."* The second was the advent of vaccinations to prevent *viral infections* such as hepatitis, measles and polio. However, there can be no vaccination for non-viral degenerative diseases such as cancer and heart disease, which are caused by nutrient deficiency. Another advance in medicine is the acceptance of the use of vitamin and mineral supplements by pregnant women. The most impressive and publicized advances were in trauma emergency room (**E.R.**) medicine, where America has become the best. Finally, the most significant advance is the change in attitude by the public who are increasingly supporting alternative medicine, and by several daring doctors who are beginning to practice such medical techniques as acupuncture, ozone, and chelation therapies.

However, for the most part, as was the case in the eighteenth and nineteenth centuries, the mistakes that the system allowed the medical and scientific authorities in America to make were continued in the twentieth century. If history is not to be repeated in the twenty-first century, the system will have to change. This can only be done by *enshrining medical freedom in the American Constitution.*

CHAPTER FOUR

THE DILEMMA OF MODERN MEDICINE

Exactly how the highly educated, intelligent, well-trained doctors and scientists of today find themselves in the same *head-in-the-sand* ostrich position that has always been adopted by their medical regulators is not difficult to understand. Both of their professions are extremely regulated and controlled by *the system*, with fatal threats for disobedience, as doctors without their licenses and scientists without their research funds find that their professions are terminated. Thus, they succumb to total control by their regulators who, because they have not learned the lessons of history, truly believe that they are doing the right thing. Besides, although they enjoy the perks, power and money, the regulators did not create the situation, but rather, they were born into it. Furthermore, the more they espouse their position, for which they earn large sums of money, *the more they believe* it, and because they are human, *the less they know* about a subject, *the more sure they are* about the position they are taking on it. These men of position and prestige all have good intentions. However, they just refuse to look at any facts that they perceive may threaten their authority.

The time of the hard-working medical practitioner is devoted and largely consumed by attending to their patients.

Both scientists and doctors are extremely sensitive to the opinions of their peers, and since *opinions are what the establishment regulates best*, the scientists and doctors become *indoctrinated* and are easy to control. However, this situation does not provide the freedom required to experiment, to be innovative, and, therefore, to discover. This is why the famous medical and scientific pioneers, who made significant discoveries, had to do so by battling the system.

History has shown that if the scientific establishment thinks enough of you to label you a "*maverick*," or if the medical establishment labels you a "*quack*" or "*snake oil salesman*," they are admitting that you are being classified in the same honorable category as: **Dalton**, the father of chemistry, who developed the atomic theory, **Dr. Ignas Semmelweis**, the father of hygiene; who fought to save the lives of thousands of women, **Louis Pasteur** and **Joseph Lister** who developed the germ theory of disease; **Albert Einstein**, a Nobel Prize winner, who was the most famous scientist of the twentieth century; **Max Planck**, the father of modern physics, who was a Nobel Prize winner, **Theodore Boverie**, the father of genetic science; **Otto Warburg**, winner of *two* Nobel Prizes; **Robert O. Becker**, one of the fathers of electro-biochemistry and a many-time contender for a Nobel Prize; **Linus Pauling**, winner of *two* Nobel Prizes; and many more men and women who are famous or are soon to be famous. Thus, *if you are criticized, shunned, and belittled by the establishment, you are following in the footsteps of many of history's most famous and respected people, who each made significant contributions to the betterment of human life.*

Thus, I am hoping that the response of the establishment to **DEATH BY DIET** will be the cries of "*quackery, charlatan*," and "*snake oil*," for then I will have succeeded in being recognized in the same category as my heroes, who are some of the best and most famous people that history has ever had to offer to the world.

18

The tragedy of the system's resistance to change is that it slows both scientific and medical advancement. The medical establishment's actions are wholeheartedly supported by the powerful drug industry, which has a vested interest in maintaining the status quo. Unfortunately, this translates into supporting human pain and suffering. History teaches us that the individual doctor and scientist *must participate* as an ignorant victim or captive of the system.

Likewise, the general public also participates as ignorant victims of the system. Many think of the medical profession in God-like terms. Each generation is impressed by the well-publicized, spectacular advances in medicine that are usually in selected, specific areas, such as surgery. For example, everyone knows – and is very proud of – the advances in American *trauma surgery*. Unfortunately, each generation believes that they know so much more than the previous generation, and believes that the previous generation had been extremely backward and handicapped in both their knowledge and capabilities. This brings up the dilemma that the *current generation*—which will be the previous generation for the next generation—*must, therefore, also be backward and handicapped* This unreasonable stance is the result of the well-planned public relations programs from the establishment of each generation that result in favorable public reaction and awe for the great scientific advances of *modern medicine.*

Despite the apparent advances in the war against disease, and there have been a few, such as polio and smallpox vaccinations, most of the wars against disease are being progressively lost. Except for viral infections, such as polio and smallpox, our worst diseases are degenerative diseases, such as diabetes, cancer and heart disease, and this is where modern medicine has totally failed. It is true that there have been some advances in helping to cure some diseases, such as heart transplants and microsurgery; however, the success of preventing degenerative disease remains at zero. Cancer, for example, was 3% at the turn of the twentieth century, 20% by 1950 and now in 2000 is at 38%. By 2020 it will reach 50%, and by the end of the century it will reach 100%. Diabetes has gone up 400% in the past two decades. We now have diseases that are ravishing our elderly – diseases that did not even exist for our grandfathers, diseases such as Alzheimer's, which currently has struck over 5 million Americans. It should also be noted – to the shame of all Americans – that our Black population has more than twice as much disease as our White population. The Blacks in Africa, who are in the sun all day long, do not have these diseases. Unfortunately the American Black does not sunbathe, and is forced to pay the ultimate price. Continuing with this horrific track record, which could bring about the end of the human race by the end of the century, is the response of the current medical establishment, while the Food and Drug Administration, responsible for protecting your health, is content to hold hands with the AMA as America drifts toward annihilation.

To put the lack of medical advances in perspective, one can imagine taking a *time trip* back in time to visit the office of the modern doctor of the last century, who was the product of the prestigious governing establishment. To your horror, a scruffy doctor who had just finished an autopsy, would enter the room and begin to treat you with dirty, unwashed hands. As painless surgery was becoming popular due to the advent of anesthesia, an abdominal complaint could result in a *go-in-blind-and-find* procedure being recommended, but only after a little bloodletting, which was also very popular at the time. Then, if you bled too much during the surgery, untyped blood could be administered. If you managed to survive this potentially lethal procedure, you might feel like screaming at the ruling establishment to *change their archaic medical procedures*. This type of blasphemy, however, may have gotten you thrown into jail, where you would most certainly have been humiliated and vilified for daring to criticize the authorities of the day.

Another enlightening *time travel trip* would be for a man or woman from the twenty-first century to visit the office of a modern twentieth-century doctor. After waiting an hour for the doctor to arrive, the time-traveler would be astounded by the *medicine-assembly-line approach*. Despite the fact that the diagnosis of the ailment would have less than a fifty percent chance of being correct, the doctor would prescribe the "*correct*" drug with confidence. No mention would be made of the preventive medicine with which the patient was so familiar. Should the diagnosis require surgery, such as the ever popular removal of the gall bladder – which was not needed, because God did not know what He was doing when he put it in the human body – the time-traveling patient from the future would be horrified by the *cut-it-out* approach. If the diagnosis were cancer, the patient would be mortified by the *cut-it-with-a-knife-and-kill-it- with-a-chemical* approach that would be supplemented with a *burn-it-out-with-radiation* procedure. Compared to the nutritional and electrophysical therapies with which the time-traveler was familiar, this establishment-endorsed medicine is barbaric. He would also be offended and astounded by the use of noxious chemicals, with their harmful side effects, that the doctor would use to reduce the pain induced by these barbaric procedures. The frustrated time-traveling patient might feel like screaming at the ruling establishment to change their *archaic medical procedures*. Unlike the nineteenth century, this type of blasphemy, however, would not get the patient thrown into jail. However, sarcastic reprimands and vilification would be in order for daring to criticize the authorities of the day.

Human nature remains the same, as history continues to repeat itself. The cycle can only be broken when there is a major change in attitude of the public brought on by education and a recognition and understanding of past events. The public must be taught that almost all grassroots practical innovators in medicine and science are rarely found in the stifling status quo establishment-oriented institutions. Rather they can usually be found toiling on a shoestring with private support from the dreamers of the world, while enduring the establishment's resistance to change.

Thus, the cause of the dilemma of modern medicine can be summed up in the quote, "*Resistance to innovation is clearly demonstrated, not by the ignorant masses, but by professionals with a vested interest in tradition and the monopoly of learning.*" (Arthur Koestler, *The Age of Velikovsky*).

CHAPTER FIVE

THE FOOD AND DRUG ADMINISTRATION

The most distressing aspect of medicine today is that the Recommended Daily Allowances (RDAs) for minerals and vitamins are rigidly adhered to even though our society is heading towards several medical disasters, as is witnessed by the staggering increase in acquired immune deficiency syndrome (AIDS) and cancer. Although medicine is winning a few battles that are highly publicized, it is losing the larger wars. For example, in the 1950s, cancer was striking one out of every four people; by the 1980s, cancer was striking one out of every three people; by the year 2010 – at the current rate of change – it is predicted that cancer will strike one out of every two people. AIDS is also skyrocketing with virtually no hope of a conventional cure. The current medical approach is to package a remedy in an expensive chemical drug, and also to maintain the almost criminally low RDAs for nutritional supplements, while totally ignoring those who advocate a nutritional approach.

In 1992, public concern was caused by legislation, *The Nutrition Labeling and Education Act*, that would put the regulation of all food, including vitamins and minerals, under the jurisdiction of the Food and Drug Administration (FDA), an agency created to maintain the quality of the food and drugs consumed by the American public. Linus Pauling, winner of two Nobel Prizes, one of which was for his research on the role of vitamins in promoting and preserving health, complained that *"Government regulators at the Food and Drug Administration remain locked in a cold war and are against vitamins when they could be encouraging education about preventing maladies."* He goes on to say that, *"It's time that the government finally caught up with a large and rapidly growing body of scientific research on nutrition."*

There is no doubt that the drug industry was eager to quash the rising popularity of the vitamin industry, which was also accompanied by the decline in popularity of orthodox medicine. The legislation would require all claims to be substantiated with scientific proof that the *unbiased* FDA would judge. The FDA can impose personal fines of up to $250,000 and business fines of up to $1,000,000. A second bill, H.R. 1662, proposed to restrict advertising and marketing of dietary supplements and nutritional products that do not conform to the nutritional labeling legislation. Wow! Talk about an incursion on your constitutional rights! And *all in the name of protecting the public.* The drug companies are obviously ecstatic with the legislation that should force the public back to the orthodox doctors dispensing their drugs. The net result will prove to be *legislated disease.*

Despite the fact that massive numbers of scientific studies over the past decades (*such as the eight-year vitamin study by the College of Medicine at the University of Chicago on 773 humans and 64 dogs which "concluded"* that a daily dosage of 10,000 IUs of vitamin D per pound of body weight was both *safe and very beneficial to health, or in other words,* a 150-pound person should consume *30 milligrams [1,500,000 IUs] of vitamin D daily, and the ten-year nutritional study by the British Medical Research Council on 5,000 men between the ages of 45 to 59, which "concluded"* that the daily consumption of milk *reduced heart*

24

disease tenfold, and the twenty-four year nutritional study by the University of Southern California on 11,384 men and women which "concluded" that not only did the daily consumption of vitamins and minerals *cut the death rate in half, but it also reduced the death rate for cancer and heart disease by tenfold*), have documented the evidence of the benefits of vitamins and minerals in preventing disease, the FDA may be duped into squeezing the vitamin industry out of business, thereby ensuring the proliferation of disease, which would be accompanied by huge increases in drug company profits. At this time, few politicians would dare to support the FDA's active incursion into the vitamin and mineral industry. The process is intended to be gradual, so as not to invoke a massive backlash from the public.

The FDA's mandate, as stated before, is to *maintain the quality* of the food and drugs consumed by the American public. Although the consumption of the artificially man-made drugs obviously requires the supervision of the medical authorities, it is difficult to understand how the consumption of natural foods, such as vitamins and minerals, would require the same supervision. Perhaps it is because the medical authorities recognize the fact that most drugs were derived from foods because they were thought to have medicinal properties to cure illness. If they believe this, then why can they not admit that food can cure illness, and, as Hippocrates most assuredly would have advised, "*Let them eat the damned garlic and onions,*" instead of the expensive white chemical drugs produced by the drug companies?

The problem with letting the medical authorities be the judges on the issue of food consumption is threefold: the first problem is that they are unqualified; a few hours' worth of training hardly puts them in the position to judge anything. True, they have some in-house experts, but these experts are under the tremendous influence of their medical masters who have to be very concerned with their second problem; that is, they are, in large part, economically dependent on the sale of drugs. Each year the drug companies make **hundreds of billions of dollars** selling doctor-prescribed drugs. The doctors charge for the prescriptions and their organizations receive other financial considerations for this service. If inexpensive food replaces most of these drugs, the financial gravy train will derail. The third problem is that both medicine and the drug companies are the biggest benefactors of ill health in America.

It is interesting to note that even though it is the publicly perceived position of the FDA that by simply eating the right foods the average person can obtain all of the vitamins and minerals required for good health, their chief, David Kessler, can be quoted as saying, "*When my wife was pregnant, I made sure she was on prenatal vitamins.*" This means that morally, if the FDA meets its publicly perceived hidden goal of removing vitamin and mineral supplements from public access, their leader could be in for a stiff fine if he continues to *practice what he does not preach*. Thus, this is another case of forcing the public to *do as I say rather than do as I do*, which is a hypocritical position to take.

What makes it more ridiculous is that doctors are trained to give this same foolish advice to their patients, causing a great deal of harm to their health. In the first place, the public should be made aware that doctors receive only *hours* of training in nutritional therapy. They are given advice by the medical authorities who are highly influenced by the drug industry, which – under no stretch of anyone's imagination – can be considered to be impartial. Can you just imagine the drug companies advising the doctors to prescribe a one-dollar piece of garlic rather than the thousand-dollar chemo drug? The other problem with their stance is that they assume that if the food is eaten, the contained nutrients will be absorbed by the body. This is not always the case. Besides, the certified nutritionists take the position that several servings of fruits and vegetables several times each day are necessary to obtain the nutrients required by the body. In one recent issue of *Reader's Digest*, seven servings were suggested as necessary. When was the last time that the average person had seven servings of fruits and vegetables in just one day? The only way that the average person is guaranteed the nutrients required for good health is to take them as food supplements. Of course, this is frowned upon by the governing establishment. The general public should not have a hard time deciding whether the scientists are correct or whether the FDA is correct.

Another problem that the general public should have with the FDA position is that their leaders acknowledge that food can cause a great deal of disease. Of course, their limited scope only allows them to think about such foods as cholesterol and fat. They then go on to quickly add that *they could not fathom any way that any food could be used for prevention or cures*. Not only is this an illogical position to take, but it ignores the fact that most drugs were developed as extracts from foodstuffs that various cultures around the world use to prevent and cure disease. It does not take much *logic* to conclude that *if diet can cause disease, then diet can prevent disease*. Although this concept is difficult for them to grasp, it is by far easier for them to live with than the concept that many cultures around the world have discovered and that will be detailed in this book, which is that *diet can also cure disease*.

If food can be shown to cure disease, the drugs, which mostly suppress symptoms of disease, will not be purchased by the public, and a large part of medicine as we know it today, and the drug companies, will be put out of business. And yet with all these problems, they claim to be unbiased. Perhaps, if they would follow the Chinese example: The doctor pays the patient if he gets sick, and if the patient stays healthy, he pays the doctor. If this were tried in America, three things would happen: First, most doctors would lose their real estate portfolios; Second, every doctor would have the prevention of disease as his major goal; and Third, doctors would acquire wealth keeping people healthy. The other obvious by-product would be the demise of the powerful drug industry as we know it today, which contributes heavily to political campaigns. Unfortunately, politicians are under tremendous pressure to maintain the status quo, making it very difficult to change the system.

This same system allows drugs to kill thousands and to inflict enormous human suffering. How many people do you know who have claimed, *"The cure was worse than the disease?"* The establishment would have you believe that these people are the victims of progress or the victims of the war against disease; however, there are those in science who are pleading that this war should be fought by using nutrition, so that the casualties and human suffering will be dramatically reduced. When was the last time that you heard or knew of anyone either dying from vitamins or complaining about the pain and side effects that they induced? The answer is probably, *"Never,"* and I am sure that the same cannot be said about the *protected and expensive drugs*. On the contrary, most of the general public has nothing but good things to say about taking vitamins and minerals.

Ironically, after expressing disapproval of the natural and nutritional vitamin and mineral supplements, the FDA has recently approved an unnatural nutrition-robbing product, known as *Olestra*. Olestra is an artificial fat with molecules too large and tightly packed for the body to break down. Thus, although it tastes like fat, it is not absorbed in the body, thereby reducing the body's fat intake. The problem is that Olestra acts like a laxative and robs the already nutrient-deficient body of even more of its crucial nutrients. Since *"nutrient deficiency"* is the cause of degenerative disease, the FDA's approval of this nutrient blocker, which will make the manufacturer billions and billions of dollars, will also have the effect of promoting even more disease and human suffering.

28

History, which has recorded many shameful acts by the Food and Drug Administration that resulted in the promotion of human disease, suffering, and death, will soon be recording another major blunder that has lead to horrific consequences, and that is the FDA approval of toxic drugs for the treatment of AIDS. In their shocking book, *Why We Will Never Win the War on AIDS*, Bryan J. Ellison and Peter H. Duesberg, systematically track the history of AIDS and the drugs approved by the FDA to treat AIDS. The book is shocking because their compelling conclusion is that *AIDS is not caused by the human immunodeficiency virus, HIV, but is actually caused by the side effects of drugs*, many of which were approved by the FDA to treat the disease. Thus, the thousands of virus hunters who have been organized to discover the magic bullet drug, have been needlessly spending billions and billions of dollars pursuing a myth, and at the cost of the research-drained budgets of other major diseases. This has lead to enormous human suffering and death and has been aggravated by the shameful approval of drugs, such as AZT (azidothymidine), by the FDA, which only increase the human suffering and death.

Peter Duesburg, a professor of molecular cell biology at the University of Berkeley and a member of the National Academy of Sciences, and the astute young scientist, Bryan Ellison, systematically and historically explain in their book how the concept of pursuing the wrong course in chasing the causes of major diseases and being wholeheartedly supported by the governing establishment, is not a new phenomenon. Interestingly, they document the history of the bacteria hunters trying to establish the bacterium that caused scurvy (which was caused by vitamin C deficiency), and the bacterium that caused beriberi, (which was caused by vitamin B-1 deficiency, commonly known as thiamin), and the bacterium that caused pellagra (which was caused by the most devastating vitamin deficiency, niacin). These bacteria hunters, much like the virus hunters of today, and their governing establishments, refused to believe that these diseases were the result of nutrient deficiency and that they could be cured simply by the consumption of the nutritious food. The result was needless human suffering and death for millions of their victims. Today, the same stubborn indifference to the treatment of disease with nutritious food exists within the pillars of power in the FDA.

Duesberg's and Ellison's arguments that HIV does not cause AIDS is overwhelming. Their position is that HIV is one of thousands of harmless viruses, many of which are carried by different individuals. They do not deny that AIDS victims are HIV positive. However, they point out that millions of people who are HIV positive have not contracted AIDS, especially on the scale predicted by the virus hunters. They note that in Africa, where there are ten times as many HIV-positive people, there are fewer cases of AIDS than in America (approximately half as many cases of AIDS in Africa) – a trend that parallels the consumption of drugs. To the layperson, this means that AIDS is 20 times more prevalent in the American HIV community. This brings up the obvious question, "*What type of virus is selective to Americans by a 20 to 1 margin?*" It does not take a rocket scientist or a virus hunter to realize that the link between HIV and AIDS is not real. However, it does result in the annual sales of billions of dollars worth of HIV- killing drugs. Duesburg points out that the gay community began consuming dozens of sex-stimulating drugs that were handed out like candy in the gay community bath houses of the late 1970s and 1980s, coinciding with the outbreak of AIDS. It is not difficult to imagine the parallel between the symptoms of drug-ravished bodies and the symptoms of AIDS. Also, except for accidental blood contamination, it is hard to conclude that an *infectious disease* would not have one teenage victim. The myth that AIDS is spreading to the

30

heterosexual community is quickly dispelled when it is learned that 96% of the women who have contracted AIDS are habitual drug users. As these women pass their drugs onto their babies, the babies suffer from the side effects of drugs. The AIDS patients who caught the HIV through blood transfusions do not suffer the major diseases found in the homosexual or injection-drug-using cases, such as Kaposi's sarcoma and dementia. Furthermore, the mid-80s prediction by the FDA of the spread of AIDS has been proven to be false. As a matter of fact, by the mid-90s, the spread of AIDS has actually diminished. The FDA will claim that their billion dollar *"drug cocktails"* are responsible, but these drugs were meant to treat AIDS, and definitely have not been proven to prevent it. Tragically, the approval by the FDA of drugs, such as AZT, that both mimic and induce the AIDS symptoms, has lead to mass confusion and fear that the harmless HIV virus will cause a plague to develop.

The overriding question is: "How could the FDA have been duped into approving toxic drugs?" AZT was developed in the 1960s as a chemotherapy drug for cancer. Technically speaking, it blocks the replication of DNA and, therefore, could block the replication of cancerous cells. The problem is, AZT also blocks the replication of healthy cells and was thereby found to be too toxic for humans. Duesburg and Ellison document in great detail in their book the sequence of events that lead the desperate virus hunters in 1986 – who had spent billions of dollars unsuccessfully trying to find a way to kill HIV – to experiment with AZT on AIDS patients. They chose 282 candidates and gave half of them AZT, and the other half a sugar placebo. Only 24 of the AZT group contracted opportunistic AIDS diseases, while 45 of the placebo group contracted the diseases. These results propelled the FDA to approve the drug AZT in 1987. Drug companies producing other chain-terminating chemicals, such as ddI and ddC, wanted in on the billion-dollar bonanzas. Given the astonishing lack of even a pretense of a controlled study, the FDA panel leaned against approval until FDA Director, David Kessler, personally intervened on behalf of the drugs and asked the board to *"be creative."* The FDA panel changed its mind and approved AZT. The results to date have been total failures. On looking back at the double-blind AZT test, shocking discrepancies were overlooked. In his book, **Poison by Prescription, the AZT Story**, Lauritsen complains that, *"The clinical trials of AZT are perhaps the sloppiest and most poorly controlled trials ever to serve as the basis for an FDA drug licensing approval."* He complains that the causes of deaths were never verified. Furthermore, the subjects in the test were not sorted according to use of drugs, and many in the placebo group were permitted to continue taking other drugs. Astonishingly, within months the death rate of the AZT group had caught up with the placebo group. It was later found that large numbers of the AZT group had discontinued the drug after only weeks due to the torturous side effects, and many of the placebo group, who experienced no side effects, knew they were on a placebo, so they illegally acquired and began taking AZT. The test study was, therefore, a farce, which has since lead to thousands of miserable deaths.

The establishment's representatives have to date failed to show up at any public forum, at which they had been scheduled to attend, to personally challenge Duesberg's findings. No doubt, at a later date, they will want to take the personal credit for rectifying the FDA's mistake of approving drugs for which they personally had grave and silent doubts.

Duesberg and Ellison point out that Americans are not the only nationality guilty of such acts of biased negligence. The Japanese viral hunters chased a disease from the late 1950s to the early 1970s that ravished hundreds of thousands of their people. The disease was known as Subacute Myelo-Optic Neuropathy, or

SMON. The disease caused intestinal problems that lead to nerve degeneration and death. Viral hunters dominated the investigative committees and even coordinated much of the work through their American counterparts. In the end, sanity prevailed, and the virus-hunting establishment was embarrassed to find out that the culprit turned out to be *a drug known as clioquinol*, which was used to treat diarrhea and dysentery. The drug was removed from public access and the epidemic was quickly over. Likewise, by removing access to FDA-approved drugs, by abstaining from the sex-stimulating drugs, and by maintaining a nutritious diet with mineral and vitamin supplements, *AIDS could be eradicated.*

On the other hand, the FDA is busy approving products – despite the risks to human health – that will generate billions of dollars for industry. For example, the FDA recently – despite the pleas from the scientific community – approved *Olestra,* a new fat substitute that should help keep the pounds off. But there is a problem, according to Meir J. Stampler, M.D., a Harvard researcher who has emerged as a leading critic of the fat. First, since Olestra passes through the body undigested, people who eat it sometimes suffer cramps and diarrhea. Second, and much more ominous, is the fact that Olestra can deplete the body of crucial fat-soluble vitamins. Stampler estimates that over the next decade, Olestra consumption could cause up to 9,800 additional cases of prostrate cancer each year, 32,00 additional cases of coronary artery disease, 7,400 additional cases of lung cancer, and 390 additional cases of macular degeneration. This will be a medical massacre.

In summary, the FDA has been guilty of ignoring the disease-preventive merits of specific foods that could have prevented epidemics, while endorsing economically lucrative toxic drugs that have been proven to cause disease. Hippocrates, the father of medicine, would have been disgusted by this performance, and so should the American public.

It is the author's hope that **DEATH BY DIET** will create opposition to any who support the position of the FDA to regulate the dispensing of food rather than to regulate the quality of food. Support should, instead, be directed to the inclusion of a multi-disciplined scientific examination of the merits of drugs and specific foods. Never again should single-minded panels, such as the bacterial hunters of the past and the virus hunters of the present, be allowed to judge the merits of a product under examination for approval. Chiropractors, acupuncturists, herbalogists, nutritionists and scientists of other disciplines should be invited to FDA panels deciding the approval of products. The enshrining of freedom of medicine in the American Constitution would end the opposition to nutritional therapy. There is no doubt in the author's mind that this *blind opposition to preventive medicine through nutritional therapy is the cause of death by diet* for the general public. Only when the public becomes enlightened, will the system change.

"There is one thing stronger than all the armies in the world; and that is an idea whose time has come" (Victor Hugo, 1802-1885).

CHAPTER SIX

THE VITAMIN ARGUMENT

Since the establishment is making such a great effort to regulate the dispensing of vitamins, the inference is that taking too many vitamins is not a healthy thing to do. There is also the inference that the vitamins themselves may be harmful and therefore they are protecting the public interest.

Of course, the majority of the public does not buy their "We are just trying to protect you!" plea. Everyone knows that their associate drug companies, which make hundreds of billions of dollars every year, are terrified by the fact that the sale of vitamins, now only in the billions of dollars each year, is beginning to encroach on their sales. If the trend were to continue into the twenty-first century, their whole market might crumble. This is a distinct possibility, as most Americans are currently vying for *alternative medicine*. In order to control this flow of change, the drug companies need to legislate control over the people's wishes. The recent establishment-supportive legislation allowing the Food and Drug Administration control over the dispensing of food is just the beginning. By doing so, establishment has taken *two steps forward* in the direction that they want to go. However, because of the popularity of vitamins and minerals, any move to exercise restrictive controls at this time would be politically unwise. It is better to do nothing and let the public forget. Although the establishment has taken *one step back* by not enforcing the legislation at this time (communist regimes always used the two-steps-forward-and-one-step-back programs as a means of suppressing personal freedom), the basic net result is *one step forward* in the direction of removal of vitamins and minerals from public access, at least, not without their written permission in the form of an expensive doctor's prescription. This draconian legislation will have the net effect of ensuring the massive and indecent profits of the drug companies in the name of protecting the public.

To add insult to injury, legislation has been passed to make it a criminal offence to make any *medical claims* without substantiated scientific proof. The judge and jurors will, of course, be those who stand to gain financially as they utter the pre-rehearsed verdict, **"GUILTY!"** Even if the large sums of money needed to satisfy the scientific requirement were met, history teaches us that logic, as has been proven by their track record in both the past and the present, will once again fail. It is a *no-win* situation where the American people – who are not allowed the freedom to speak their opinion – are the biggest losers. Once again the establishment will be able to save the public from *the medical charlatans and their quackery*.

The problem with all this is that it has been done based on the assumption that the medical authorities are right, and that the perpetuated myth that *vitamins could be bad for your health* is true. But, as a careful examination of medical history and the scientific facts will show, this is simply not the case.

First let us examine the "*too much*" theory. Sure there are some limited recent studies that may suggest that consumption of too many vitamins may have detrimental effects, but then the argument of *too much of anything* usually has scientific merit.

The problem is that all consumables fall into the **too much** category. The argument against removing the offending consumable becomes ridiculous. For example, too much salt—which is essential for life—could kill you. Should salt be removed by the regulators? Also, since you could drown from a glass of water, should the regulators ban drinking water? The list of *"too much"* consumables is endless. Of course, the regulators would never be foolish enough to ban any of the consumables, including vitamins. Their intent is to reduce and economically control their use.

Where did the concept of *"too many"* vitamins originally come from? The answer lies in the history of the beginning of the twentieth century, when the public found that vitamins had benefits to human health and began to consume them in earnest. Vitamins are natural organic substances which, with only minute amounts, encourage normal biological reactions to both occur and occur at a fast rate, were discovered and found to have benefits to human health. The first problem was that they were not easily manufactured in a pure form, and the impurities could have some side effects. Because of the deemed health benefits, the side effects were ignored, just as they are with the drugs of today (if side effects were the bases of removing consumables from the market, then there would virtually be almost no drugs today). These benefits caused the public to use the logic that *if one pill a day is good for you, then ten pills must be ten times as good for you.*

Thus, consumption went up dramatically. By the 1920s, people were consuming millions (mega) of international units (IUs) of vitamins daily and hence the name **megavitamins** was coined. Even though dramatic beneficial medical claims were common, the establishment reasoned that, because the use of **mega** amounts of anything is not natural, megavitamins must be detrimental to human health. The problem they had with this position is that consumption of megavitamins had become so popular that the establishment dared not intervene. Also, the public began staying away from hospitals and doctors in droves, claiming all kinds of *magical cures*. The establishment was there by confronted with its worst dilemma since the inception of the AMA back in 1839.

Then, to their delight, someone who could be documented finally did take *too much* of a vitamin. In fact it was a group of people: *six medical students* became very sick. They had taken *large mega* (this sounds redundant but actually will be understood not to be, once the word *megavitamin* has been technically defined) *doses* of vitamin D, (and not common table salt which would have had the same effect) and had become acutely sick. The hiding-in-waiting medical authorities launched into action, not only banning the offending vitamin, but also removing all the existing vitamins from the sales shelves. Thus, the modern medicine of the time had been saved, at least from competition.

The resulting public outcry forced an investigation into the matter. The public demanded a thorough investigation to determine if large doses of vitamin D were truly toxic and whether the evidence, which they believed was fabricated by the medical establishment, had any real scientific merit. Thus, in 1929, with the public looking on, the College of Medicine (University of Chicago) began an extensive study that included 773 human subjects and 64 dogs.

The study was carried out by the scientific elite of the day: I.E. Streck, M.D.; H. Deutch, A.B.; C.I. Reed, PhD; and H.C. Struck, PhD. By the time the public had lost interest, they concluded in 1937 that *"Humans and dogs generally survive the daily administration of 20,000 international units (IUs) per kilogram of body weight."* This means that a 110-pound woman

38

could take 1,000,000 IUs each day without any serious consequences. This raises the question, *"Where did the current Recommended Daily Allowance (RDA) of 400 IUs come from?"* especially as this study has been backed up by other extensive studies. It also brings up the question, *"Why are doctors today so adamant about **the harm vitamin D can cause?**"* when comprehensive scientific studies, such as this one carried out by the University of Chicago, *have concluded just the opposite.*

It was fortunate for the medical authorities that the general public of the time was asleep or preoccupied by Hitler's activities in Europe, as they quietly responded by *maintaining the low-dose recommendation,* that is, except for doctors who began prescribing *drugs* such as *Dalsol, Deltalin, and Drisdol* for their arthritis patients. These drugs *contained large doses of vitamin D as the active ingredient* and the patients responded by extolling the virtues of these modern drugs. The study also concluded that many of the medical benefit claims made by the public were valid. This makes one wonder just *how large* was the dosage that made the medical students sick?

The study of the potential of megavitamins to damage human health was not over. In the 1940s, the results of a massive study done at the Louisiana State University entitled, *Comparative Therapeutic Value and Toxicity of Various Types of Vitamin D* (C. Reynolds, M.D.) also re-evaluated the University of Chicago 1937 study and suggested that the toxicity of some of the massive doses given to the dogs may have been due to the *chemical impurities* in the vitamins rather than the vitamins themselves.

The Louisiana State University study suggests that *doses of vitamin D in the millions of IUs per day are quite safe.* With this in mind, it is important to understand just what an international unit means. It takes 40,000 IUs of vitamin D to make just one milligram, or one thousandth of a gram, or two millionths of a pound. A mega dose of 1,000,000 IUs is therefore only 25 milligrams – about the size of a few grains of salt. One wonders what all the fuss was about and how the medical establishment could have the public brainwashed into believing that *mega means bad and too much vitamin may be harmful to your health*.

Another vitamin that Americans have been caused to become concerned about is vitamin A. Its ridiculously low RDA is 5,000 IUs. A person eating a modest meal of carrots and liver consumes at least 1,000,000 IUs of vitamin A, and he does it without a doctor's prescription. Spinach, sweet peas, potatoes, red peppers and dried apricots would also be disallowed from the doctor's prescription if the FDA ever is allowed to enforce the RDAs. If vitamin A is so abundant in common food then how could the medical authorities convince the doctors to warn the public about the dangers of taking *too much* and that it could be *poisonous?*

The answer most frequently cited is that eating polar bear livers, which contain as much as 8,000,000 IUs of vitamin A, was fatal for the early arctic explorers. My God! When was the last time that you ate polar bear liver? The tragedy behind this ridiculous stance is that it is based on misinformation. To begin with, the early explorers did not die from eating the polar bear liver, but rather became sick, suffering from dermatitis and defoliation, which are symptoms of cadmium metal poisoning. In the late 1980s, a team of Swedish scientists discovered that polar bear liver adsorbs large amounts of cadmium metal found in the arctic water. Thus, the ailments of the early explorers were caused by the cadmium in the polar bear liver, and not the large amount of vitamin A. However, one has to wonder what the effects of constantly eating 1,600 times the recommended daily allowance of vitamin A would be on your health, as *too much* of anything cannot be good for your health.

The other tragedy caused by this stance is that it has been found, by several recent scientific studies, that eating 20 times the RDA of vitamin A really does *inhibit cancer.* In 1993, in a medical trial in Linxian, China, Chinese scientists, along with scientists from the American National Cancer Institute, established that beta-carotene, a chemical cousin of vitamin A, in combination with vitamin E and selenium, reduces deaths from cancer. This supports the work done by medical researchers at the beginning of the century who found that a severe lack of vitamin A caused stomach cancer in rats. The Chinese took the vitamins and mineral as a food supplement, but because of the American medical system, the National Cancer Institute scientists have rushed home *"to study drugs that might achieve the same effect."* In other words, *American scientists have found a nutritional and inexpensive way to treat cancer, but prefer instead to try to develop an expensive chemical for the drug companies.* Once again I am sure that Hippocrates is screaming from his grave, "Why don't you just let them eat the damned food?"

Vitamin A is such a critical food that it is important to understand some of its other health benefits. The ancient Egyptians squeezed the juice from livers to treat night blindness and other eye disorders. This *strong medicine* is known today as vitamin A or retinol. Now, in the twentieth century, most people in the West do not experience severe vitamin A deficiency, as they acquire some of the vitamin in the foods they eat. Unfortunately, in poor countries, it is estimated that 500,000 children go blind each year for lack of vitamin A. Scientists in India recently found that weekly vitamin A supplements for school children cut deaths from disease by more than half. ("The A Team" Tim Beardsley, February 1991, *Scientific American*).

Thus, by examining the scientific history of the two vitamins in question, it has been shown that their RDAs are not only ridiculously low, but almost criminally irresponsible. An examination of each of the other vitamins would prove the same conclusion. For example, only 1,200 IUs, or 60 milligrams of vitamin C is recommended, and yet Linus Pauling, who won a Nobel Prize for his studies on vitamin C, recommends 100,000 IUs (5,000 milligrams) per day. Merv Griffin tells his audience that he takes 50,000 IUs. every day and has not had a cold for many years. If the FDA enforces the gag rule on vitamin claims, I wonder if they, along with somebody else's army, are planning to arrest Mr.Griffin.

As the sunshine on the skin of a man in a bathing suit can cause the production of about 20,000 IUs of vitamin D each hour, the FDA agents will soon be storming the beaches to arrest those who have exposed themselves to more than 2 minutes or 400 IUs. Also arrested on the beach will be the child who exceeded his allowable vitamin C by taking a second glass of orange juice. Although the situations as described are laughable, and probably will never happen, the current law of the land does give the FDA the power to make it happen. The legislators who passed the bill obviously left their calculators at home or were incapable of using them, as their arms and minds had been *twisted by the drug lobby*.

All this evidence leads one to question how the powers that be came up with their ridiculously low recommendations. For most Americans, the daily amounts of vitamins contained in the foods they eat are much higher than the RDAs. For other Americans, the RDAs either match or are higher than their daily intake. Science shows us that these will be the sick Americans. The authorities are often coming up with small studies to validify their numbers, but they have to do this by ignoring the massive studies of the past, and basic science. Thus, *the RDAs can be described as what the average sick American eats.*

CHAPTER SEVEN

THE MINERAL ARGUMENT

The establishment is also taking pains and making a great effort to **regulate the dispensing of minerals**. Although they are much more liberal in their attitude towards minerals than vitamins, unjustified paranoia still prevails. The inference is the same as their inference on vitamins: taking too many minerals is not a healthy thing to do. There is also the *"inference"* that certain minerals may be harmful, and therefore, they are protecting the public interest.

Of course, as is the case with vitamins, the majority of the public does not buy their, *"We are just trying to protect you!"* plea. Everyone knows that their associate drug companies stand to lose billions of dollars when the minerals are proven to have health benefits. The recent legislation allowing the Food and Drug Administration's control over the dispensing of food is aimed at mineral supplements. The basic net result will be to require an expensive doctor's prescription in order to purchase mineral supplements. The net effect will be increased disease, ensuring the massive and **indecent profits** of the drug companies in the name of protecting the public.

The difference between the establishment's position on vitamin and mineral supplements is that there is so much *overwhelming scientific support* for the benefits of minerals, much of which will be discussed in subsequent chapters, that the establishment is beginning to endorse their moderate use. Thus, it has become extremely important to the establishment to have legislation in place providing controls before their use becomes a phenomenon that could jeopardize the drug industry profits. Once again, all this has been done based on the assumption that the medical authorities are right that too much of the *good minerals* is bad for you. But, just as the careful examination of medical history and the scientific facts showed that the establishment *was wrong about vitamins, the same examination proves that they are also wrong about minerals*, especially common salt.

Currently, 50% of Americans consume some minerals and vitamin supplements: About 25% consume both of them on a daily basis. A 24-year study of 11,384 people by Professor James E. Enstrom of the University of Southern California found that taking *vitamins and supplements cut the death rate in half.* Even more astonishing was the fact that deaths from cancers and heart disease for those taking the daily supplements was less than 10% of those who did not take the supplements. This study by respected scientists at a prestigious institute of learning, of large numbers of people over a long time, will be an excellent candidate for the AMA's wastebasket, as it withholds funding for the studies, rather than verify the results that are crucial to the health of America. The medical establishment will demand more proof as they watch Americans die.

A recent four-year study by the prestigious Albert Einstein College of Medicine (done in association with the prestigious Cornell University Medical College) on 1,900 men with high blood pressure, concluded that high blood pressure patients who ate less than five grams of salt a day had **more than four times as many heart attacks** as those who consumed over ten grams a day. Although a *"tremendous"* increase in salt can lead to a *"small"* increase in blood pressure, low sodium causes the level of renin hormone, secreted by the kidneys, in the blood to go up, and renin is found in high levels of patients with high blood pressure.

The party-line trace quantities of nutrients that doctors recommend to their patients have been *arbitrarily* determined by the medical authorities, and have no scientific merit. In fact, Recommended Daily Allowances (RDAs) of vitamins and minerals were based on the amounts of these nutrients already present in the diet of the typical, *"already sick"* American. Even this approach was inaccurately assessed. For example, they recommended only *5,000 IUs* (international units) *of vitamin A daily.* To show how ridiculously low an intake of 5,000 IUs really is: a man eating a modest meal of carrots and liver consumes 100,000 IUs and without a doctor's prescription! Spinach, sweet potatoes, red peppers, and dried apricots would also be disallowed from the doctor's prescribed meal. Warnings are also given that *"vitamin A is poisonous*, because eating *polar bear livers*, an especially rich source (over 8,000,000 IUs of vitamin A per pound), *"can be fatal*," as was reported in February 1991, (*Scientific American*, "The A Team" by T. Beardsley). Of course, eating *1,600 times* the recommended daily dose of *anything* – including water – could be hazardous to your health. Contrary to some reports, the early explorers *did not die* from eating polar bear livers, but rather, they experienced exfoliative dermatitis and loss of hair. It is also interesting to note that in 1988, a Swedish team of scientists discovered that the polar bear and seal livers tended to accumulate cadmium metal from the polar waters. The symptoms for *cadmium poisoning* are the same as experienced by the early explorers, exfoliative dermatitis and loss of hair. Vitamin A has also been shown by several scientific studies to *inhibit cancer*, the amount necessary, however, is *20 times* the Recommended Daily Allowance ("Diet and Cancer," Lenard A. Cohen, *Scientific American*, November 1987). Despite these scientific facts, most doctors remain erroneously convinced that vitamin A in large amounts is toxic.

To most people, the word calcium is synonymous with mineral supplements. Numerous food advertisements extol the virtues of the calcium to be found in their products. The **Tums**® claim to be a nutritional antacid is technically correct, due to its high calcium content. These advertisers make special efforts to represent their product in terms of fractions of RDAs, so as not to offend the authorities and so that the public, many of whom believe in the validity of the RDAs, will not become afraid of ill health caused by excess consumption.

Their concern is well-founded, as the public has become sensitized by the constant concerns expressed by their doctors. Because of the *overwhelming evidence* provided in *thousands of scientific publications* each year, most of these doctors now believe in the benefits of calcium consumption in the treatment of bone disease, such as osteoporosis. However, when these same doctors discover calcium buildup in the joints of some patients, they warn these people to avoid the consumption of calcium. They have been incorrectly taught to reason that the reduction in the consumption of calcium will result in a reduction in the calcium buildup in the joints. Although this argument may have a little merit, the effect of such actions on the patient's health could be catastrophic.

The most important question to ask is, "*Why is the calcium buildup in the joints in the first place?*" The answer is that these patients are calcium deficient. In order to acquire the required calcium for the body's numerous biological functions, the body's parathyroid hormones oversee the removal of some calcium from the body's *bone bank*. When the calcium deficiency is severe, the removal of calcium from the bones is extensive. This results in a dramatically weakened and sagging architectural structure. The body – which always knows best – adapts to the situation by physically reducing movement with a little pain, calcium deposits and spurs in the joints, thereby minimizing bone breaks. The misinformed doctor's recommendation to reduce calcium will only serve to aggravate and prolong the problem, as the body is desperate for more calcium to be returned to its bone bank, and in amounts substantially higher than the RDA.

Although there is enormous scientific evidence on the importance to human health of other minerals, such as potassium, magnesium and sodium, substantial amounts of calcium are also considered to be critical to human health. The following are but a few of the thousands of such statements being made by world-renowned medical researchers:

"Calcium deficiency is the universal property of all cancer cells." (***The Role of Calcium in Biological Systems***, Volume I, 1985, CRC Press Inc.)

"The rise in calcium ions is indispensable for cell proliferation (DNA synthesis)," ***Calcium and the Cell*** (L.K. Defize, and S.W. Delaat, 1986, Wiley.)

"The prime period of human life could be extended by a moderate increase in calcium in the diet," Dr. Henry C. Sherman in the book ***How a Mineral Can Vitalize Your Health***, by Dr. James K. Van Fleet (1980, Parker Publishing.)

"The calcium ion regulation of intracellular messages has broad implications in the treatment of disease," (**"The Calcium Signal,"** Ernesto Carafoli and John T. Penniston, November 1987, *Scientific American.)*

"Considering the wide variety of calcium binding proteins in the cell, the potential targets of calcium related disorders are enormous." (***Calcium Binding Proteins***, Marvin P. Thompson, 1988, CRC Press.)

Other vitamins, such as vitamin D, were also considered to be *dangerous* – except in exceedingly low dosage – by the medical authorities. Only 400 IUs were allowed, this despite the fact that the human body can generate up to 10,000 IUs on a good sunny day at the beach. Only 1,200 IUs or 60 milligrams of vitamin C are recommended; this despite the fact that you exceed your daily dose with one glass of orange juice. Nobel Prize winner, Dr. Linus Pauling recommended up to 5,000 milligrams (100,000 IUs) daily, while Merv Griffin tells his audience that he takes 2,500 milligrams (50,000 IUs) daily and has not had a cold for many years.

The experts say calcium is crucial in the prevention of cancer, in DNA synthesis, in extending life and in the treatment and prevention of disease. It is therefore important, not only to be consumed in healthy amounts, but also to be absorbed into the body, and therein lies the major problem with RDAs. Even if a vitamin or mineral RDA is within a reasonable scientific level, consumption does not always translate into absorption by the body. That is why the doctor who tells his patients that, "You can get all the nutrients you need *by eating the right foods*," is the doctor who does not know what he is "biochemically." Unfortunately, the doctor is only telling you what he was told to tell you by those with a vested interest, the AMA/FDA/Drug Industry coalition, in keeping you sick. The bottom line is that if the nutrient is not in the soil, as has been concluded by Senate investigations, then it is impossible for it to be in the plants that grow in the soil. Also, the consumption of some foods interferes with the absorption of other crucial nutrients. For example, the phosphates found naturally in meat or artificially put into carbonated drinks (to keep your teeth from disintegrating) combine with the digested calcium in your stomach to form a bony precipitate which then is expelled by the body. This precipitous sludge causes other nutrients to precipitate, resulting in a substantial loss of nutrients by the body. Thus soda pop, such as Coke, in reality, will do long-term damage to your health, and most of the Pepsi® generation is already filling our hospital beds. It should also be noted that even when phosphates are not present, the lack of vitamin D in the small intestine – which is very common in America – also dramatically reduces the absorption of ionized calcium and other ionized mineral nutrients that are crucial to good health. Despite the massive scientific information available on the health benefits of vitamin D, the medical establishment's literature is full of articles warning the doctors that vitamin D "may" be or "could" be toxic.

As a result, despite all this massive scientific evidence, the average doctor still believes the myth of vitamin D toxicity. For example, it was recently brought to my attention by medical pioneer, Carl Taylor, M.D. from Edmonton, Canada that the medical community was constantly being bombarded with technical information *suggesting* that vitamin D was toxic. Dr. Taylor sent me an article as an example, entitled, *"A Brief History of Vitamin D Toxicity"* (*Journal of Applied Nutrition*, Volume 49, Numbers 1& 2, 1997, James C. Moon, Ph.D., FACN, CNS.)

Although I found the article to be a treasure trove of information, the article was basically "misinformation" as the only proof presented about the toxicity of vitamin D was in reality *"toxicity by insinuation."* Nowhere did the article provide proof or provide statements on vitamin D toxicity such as *"concludes that ..."* Instead, referring to vitamin D toxicity, it used words such as *"suggests that ..."*, *"may lead to ..."* and *"may result in ..."* These words by themselves demonstrate the lack of proof in this article of the toxicity of vitamin D. By using the phrase "excessive vitamin D *may lead to hypercalcemia*," vitamin D is then held responsible for the damage to health caused by hypercalcemia, when in fact, just the opposite is true. High serum calcium levels are a direct result of decalcification of the bones for the purpose of supplying calcium to the organs that are desperate for calcium. It is also due to a lack of sunshine, resulting in low calcium-regulating calcitonin production, and calcium-storage inisotol triphosphate production. Calcium deficiency due to lack of calcium in the diet, along with lack of exposure to sunshine, are responsible for hypercalcemia. Vitamin D produced by sunshine, allows the body to absorb large quantities of calcium and therefore helps to prevent hypercalcemia. Also, the sunshine that produces the vitamin D also causes the pituitary gland to instruct the parathyroid gland to produce the hormone calcitonin, which prevents the decalcification of the bones. Thus, vitamin D *actually prevents the health problems it is accused of causing.* The scientific studies that "suggested" otherwise did not include the other numerous health factors that play a major role in hypercalcemia. None of these studies meet the basic requirement of being *"multi year, phase 1, 2 and 3, double-blind, and massive studies done on large numbers of individuals,"* that are requirements to scientifically determine toxicity.

Typical of articles attempting to perpetuate the myth that God's nutrient, vitamin D, is toxic, the article not only provides misinformation, it also uses arguments that are not true. For example, it states "there have been no systematic studies to determine vitamin D toxicity for humans." In the previous pages I have provided 12 such studies, *"all"* of which *conclude that vitamin D is not toxic.* Many of these were ten-year studies done on hundreds of animals and humans. Studies that were carried out by our best scientists and doctors at our best scientific research establishments. For example, the Streck Report of 1937, *"Further Studies on Intoxification With Vitamin D,"* which was done at the University of Chicago Medical Facility and took dozens of doctors and scientists nine years to complete, concluded that they found large doses of vitamin D to be non-toxic and, because of the correlation of their animal studies to their human studies, they concluded that *"the burden of proof rests with those who claim the undesirability of vitamin D therapy."* This study was followed up by other massive studies which all concluded the "non-toxicity of vitamin D."

50

Finally, this article did provide information that proved that vitamin D, in amounts such as 1,200 IUs and 2,000 IUs, which they claimed were toxic—just simply could not possibly be toxic. It is simple because all one has to do is apply eighth grade math to the numbers provided in the article. The article refers to a paper, **"Cholecalciferol Production"** by P.C. Beadle, where Beadle measured the vitamin D production in the epidermis (skin) to be 163 IUs per square centimeter in *light skin* per day, and 69 IUs per square centimeter in *dark skin* per day. The human body has about 20 square feet of skin or 18,600 square centimeters. This means that the human body can produce over *3,000,000 IUs of non toxic vitamin D per day*. Also, the article suggests that 30 minutes of sunshine per week produces enough vitamin D for the human body. Assuming this to be true, and also assuming that there is 12 hours of sunlight per day, the amount of vitamin D produced in 30 minutes is 128,000 IUs, which calculates to 18,300 IU per day. This means that they are advising that "18,300 IUs of vitamin D are required by the human body per day" (which this author wholeheartedly supports), while saying at the same time that 1,200 IUs "may be toxic." Which is it, 18,000 or 1,200? The latter is ludicrous as the healthiest people in the world—the Hunzas in Pakistan, the Bamas in China, the Georgians in Russia, the Titicacas in Peru and the Okinawans in Japan, all of whom have virtually no diseases, all get about 7 hours of sunshine each day and therefore produce about 500,000 IUs of Vitamin D each day (their skin is dark). Thus, the logic of the PhDs who apparently cannot calculate, lies in the ruins of eighth grade math.

Other interesting studies have been done. *The Lancet*, (Garland et al, February 9, 1985 issue) reported that a long study had shown that men with the highest vitamin D in the blood had 1.42% colon cancer whereas those with the lowest had 3.89% (or 273% more cancer). *The Lancet* (Garland et al, November 18, 1989 issue) reported a study of 25,000 in Maryland that showed that there were

80% more colon cancers in the fifth of the population with the lowest Vitamin D in the blood. In a report from England, (*The Lancet,* March 23, 1991), stated that 3 of 14 women who were treated with topical vitamin D experienced a reduction of 50% in their malignant breast tumors. A report in *Cancer* (70, 1992, pp 2861-9) by C.C. Hanchette and G.G. Schartz entitled,*"Geographic Patterns of Prostate Cancer Mortality, Evidence for Protective Effect of Ultraviolet Radiation"* notes that areas in northern latitudes, such as Iceland, Denmark and Sweden have far more prostate cancers than found in areas of more intense sunlight. A report from M. Frydenburg of the Urology Department in the Royal Melbourne Hospital in *Cancer Forum* (Vol. 19, No 1, March 1995, pp 15-18) states that high vitamin D in the blood may be protective for prostate cancer.

It should also be remembered that the RDA of vitamin D is only 400 IUs (or fewer than 0.01 milligrams), and the successful biological absorption function of the mineral nutrients requires many thousands of IUs. Thus, much of the 1,400 milligrams (RDA) of calcium that would be consumed *readily passes through the body*. This means that even if the current RDAs are adhered to, healthy nutrient absorption is destined to fail. This gradually leads to disease, and is therefore currently the main cause resulting in *death by diet*.

In conclusion, medical doctors are reading and believing the thesis that vitamin D is toxic, and as a result are *"perpetuating disease."* Ironically, I know medical doctors who claim to have treated patients suffering from vitamin D toxicity. This only proves to demonstrate the medical fact that *"at least 50% of all medical diagnoses are incorrect."* The use of vitamin D with calcium supplementation could make a major impact on the war against disease. All be to read: **Death By Diet.**

CHAPTER EIGHT

THE BODY'S FLUIDS

In the previous chapters, the important role that the mineral and vitamin supplements have on human health has been established. There is no doubt that today the general public believes that vitamin and mineral supplements provide some benefit to human health. What they do not know is just how important these benefits are to their very survival. They also do not know how these supplements *do what they do*.

The common denominator in the benefits of nutrients to human health is *the body's fluids*, which act as the transportation medium for the delivery of the nutrients to the cells that make up the human body, and the expulsion of toxins from the body. These same fluids carry the nutrients inside the cells and participate in many of the body's biochemical reactions. All of these fluids are interdependent and if the fluid system becomes restricted or impaired in any way, the result can be disastrous to human health.

There are some basic properties of the body's fluids that are important for the general public to understand. The first and most obvious is that all of the body's fluids have many things in common: they are all in the same body, they are all totally dependent on each other, and certain fluids are by-products of other fluids. This may all seem very logical to you, but you would be surprised at how many doctors have been told, *"the saliva has nothing to do with the blood."* As far as this example is concerned, nothing could be farther from the truth, and nothing could have a more profound impact on human health than the perpetuation of such misinformation. The human body produces up to seven quarts of saliva daily. That's almost two gallons, and would require a huge saliva pouch, except that saliva is produced upon demand. There are three glands in the mouth, which extract fluids from the blood, producing the saliva. As many nutrients are more crucial to the blood than to the saliva—calcium for example— to keep the blood alkaline and full of oxygen, the blood will retain these nutrients, resulting in a deficiency of the nutrient in the saliva. Fortunately, this deficiency can be readily measured with an inexpensive piece of pH paper. Thus, the blood is definitely biologically connected with saliva despite the doctor's misconception.

Except for the fluids entering the body in the stomach, and the fluids leaving the body in the kidneys and colon, *all of the body's fluids are alkaline*, or rather, they are supposed to be to maintain good health. In other words, they are not supposed to be acidic. As a matter of fact, they are all supposed to be at the same slightly alkaline level: a pH measurement of 7.4. Just go to the library and you will find that a host of medical and biochemical books back up this claim. This does not help the layperson to understand fluids, as I am sure that there are many who do not have a clue what the letters "pH" mean.

In as simple terms as I can give you, the pH is the logarithmic measurement of the level of acidity, which is the measurement of hydrogen ions in a fluid. *"Logarithmic"* simply means that each change of one unit is a difference of tenfold. Now here comes the main problem: zero does not mean zero acid, as a pH of 7.0 is neutral (with no acid or no alkali). Anything above 7.0 is alkaline, and anything below is acidic. The higher above a pH of 7.0, the more alkali ions the fluid contains. Likewise, the farther below 7.0 the pH is measured, the more acid ions the fluid contains. For example, a pH of 3.0 would be ten times as acidic as a pH of 4.0 (remember that the readings are logarithmic, and each change of one full unit is tenfold). Thus, a reading of 3.0 is one hundred times more acidic than a reading of 5.0, and a reading of 4.0 is one thousand times more acidic than a pH of 7.0. The last example is important to remember, as it will prove to be pertinent to those who have a terminal degenerative disease. The best way to learn about the pH scale is to study the following table.

TABLE 1: pH

	pH Value	Ratio of (H)+ Concentration
	0	10,000,000
	1	1,000,000
Excess of (H)+ Ions	2	100,000
	3	10,000
Acid Side	4	1,000
	5	100
	6	10
⟶ Neutrality ⟶	7	— Neutrality ⟶
	8	10
	9	100
Alkali Side	10	1,000
	11	10,000
Excess of (OH)- Ions	12	100,000
	13	1,000,000
	14	10,000,000

Ratio of (OH)- Concentration

The most important thing to remember about the pH is that healthy body fluids are supposed to be a slightly alkaline pH 7.4, except for excreted fluids, which are slightly acidic—between 5.0 and 6.5—and the stomach fluids, which can be highly acidic, below a pH of 1.0. All other fluids are alkaline, as *most generic disease is caused by acidosis*. Another important fact to remember is that all of the fluids are interdependent—the body balances the contents to obtain the best biological values.

This last statement leads us to the most controversial part: *the state of your health is reflected by the state of your acidosis* or lack of it. Even more controversial is the fact that your *acidosis* is reflected by *the pH or acid level* of your saliva. Now, I suppose that you are thinking that you are going to need a piece of scientific equipment called a pH meter to measure your saliva. Well, you are wrong! You can do it yourself, and it is very simple. First, you must remember that *you are measuring the pH of your saliva, and not the food in your mouth*. Also remember that your body produces gallons of saliva every day and delivers it to your mouth through two glands under your tongue. You are trying to measure the saliva in your body and therefore must draw fresh saliva into the mouth. It is best if this is done several times before the test. Once you have done this, simply spit on a small strip of pH paper. The paper will immediately change color *reflecting your pH and your state of health*. The cost is about a penny.

By now, I'm sure that the authorities are screaming that I have made a *medical claim*, and that I am recommending that the patient doctor himself or herself. Of course, that is ridiculous, as all that I have done is state scientific facts, with which, of course, they will never agree, regardless of the evidence. I have probably also committed a transgression by informing the public that the test is both simple and that they can do it themselves. The recommendation of taking one's temperature as a measure of one's state of health—which is the same principle—I am sure will not cause the medical uproar that the *penny pH test* will cause.

The blind argument that something so simple and so inexpensive could not possibly work should fuel the cries of "*quackery,*" to which I point out that millions had to die because their predecessors thought that something as simple as the washing of hands could not possibly have such a profound effect on your health. Anyway, the critics are wrong, as anybody with five cents (five tests) worth of pH paper will soon find out. The pH paper can be purchased for a few dollars for a 25-foot roll—less than a penny per test—from some pharmacies and scientific supply companies.

Once the public knows that the pH of healthy body fluids is supposed to be 7.4, the question then becomes, "*Why?*" And more important, "*How do I maintain a pH of 7.4?*" Of course, with the explanation of why, the how—currently not well understood by medical experts—will become very important.

To begin with, everyone in the scientific and medical professions knows that the pH of the blood is supposed to be 7.4. In fact, this pH is so critical that a slight change—just over one tenth of a unit of measurement (0.1)—will cause instant death (within minutes). The human body is also well aware of this fact, and therefore, in His wisdom, God created *two systems* in order to maintain this pH: the main system is a *biochemical buffering system* that works extremely well—as long as ample mineral nutrients exist in the body (such as the young and healthy); the second system is a unique method of the body *robbing-the-Peter-fluid-to-pay-the-Paul-fluid*. The latter system is only necessary when the body is experiencing a mineral deficiency (such as the elderly, the sick, and those who do not take mineral supplements).

Thus, when the blood pH level begins to drop, the body immediately supplies it with mineral nutrients. If the body is mineral deficient, it quickly robs the required mineral nutrients from the important, but *less critical*, saliva. Most of the mineral nutrients are in the form of alkaline salts, which are derived from the mineral nutrients that the body had expected us to consume and replenish. Therefore, due to the removal of alkaline nutrients from the saliva, the acid level goes up, meaning that its pH drops below the natural 7.4.

To test this theory, as the author has done thousands of times, first test the saliva pH of healthy children, and then test the pH of your friends. The children and friends who are obviously *healthy will be bright blue, at a pH of 7.5*. This category is your goal, as the body contains enough mineral nutrient that it does not have to rob Peter to pay Paul. Your friends who are not feeling well or who are experiencing some minor health problems will be *green, at a pH of 6.0 to 6.5*. In this category, you may likely be in the stage of developing a disease, as your body has found it necessary to begin robbing Peter to pay Paul. Your friends who have major health problems will be *yellow–green, at a pH of 5.0 to 6.0* . This category means that you already have a major disease, such as diabetes, arthritis, or heart disease, even though the symptoms may not have manifested themselves. Unfortunately, your friends who have a terminal health disease will be *bright yellow, at a pH of 4.5 to 5.0*. This last category includes diseases such as cancer and AIDS in their later stages. It is important to remember that the pH measurements that you have just taken are logarithmic, or in other words, your terminal friend with the pH of 4.5 is *1,000 times more acidic* than your healthy friend with a pH of 7.5. After just a few minutes of testing everyone's saliva pH, you will be convinced at just how well this simple and inexpensive test works.

So convinced was one group of nurses at a major hospital, that they had posted a chart on a bulletin board of all the nurses' states of health versus their saliva pH. As they were explaining to me how amazed they were at the accuracy of the test, two doctors walked by and one pointed at me and said in a loud, condescending voice, "*There's that calcium nutrition nut.*" The head nurse quickly took me aside and responded, "*Don't listen to them; a lot of people who do, end up in **early graves**.*" And, before I could say anything, one of three, sweet elderly ladies standing nearby in white gowns replied, "*We have been eagerly listening to what you have been saying about the saliva test, and as far as we are concerned, we don't care what those doctors think. We would like you to take all of our pHs.*" I smiled at them and responded, "Of course," and I turned to get a roll of pH paper out of my brief case. I could hear the sounds of metal rollers, as someone was obviously opening a large curtain. As I turned back around, there stood a room full of smiling, white-gowned, elderly and obviously sick patients. I tried not to gasp, as all tested bright yellow, 1,000 times more acidic than normal healthy people. Seeing my dismay, they all tried to comfort me. The nurses later informed me that I was standing in the *terminal cancer ward*.

When giving talks on the subject of America's trend of *death by diet*, I always try to have pH paper readily available to all those listening. The trick to convincing everyone about the authenticity of the saliva pH test is to have everyone take the test at the same time. This means that after each person looks at his or her own colored pH paper, the temptation to look at the result of the closest person is just too great. As a matter of fact, the room is usually abuzz with everyone comparing their test results. As those who are sick usually know it, and those who are healthy also know it, it does not take long for everyone to agree that the test worked. But some always have a hard time admitting that something so simple could possibly work on something as important to them as their own state of health. A few diehards will continue to refuse to believe the results until they are told by their doctors to do so.

Unfortunately for them, the system does not allow orthodox doctors to practice this type of preventive medicine. One adventurous doctor recently told me, "*After seeing 60 patients today I did not find one that had a **pH of over 6.5**.*" He then questioned, "*Are you sure that the saliva pH test really works?*" I responded that he already had proven that it worked, as, "*Your patients went to see you, not because they were a healthy blue, but because they were a sick green.*" After quickly testing and discovering that his healthy children and healthy self were all a bright blue 7.5 pH, subdued, he responded, "***My God! You will put us out of business!***"

Now that you have been introduced to the saliva test, it is time to answer the question of, "***How do I attain healthy alkaline saliva?***" It is first necessary to understand a little about the chemistry of the body fluids so that you will understand what causes the pH to become acidic in the first place. I will try to make the explanation as simple as possible and only use terms that the layperson will understand.

As was previously mentioned, the stomach is very acidic. In fact, it can have a pH of less than 1.0, which (see the pH Table) you can see is ***over 1,000,000 times the acidity level of healthy saliva at a pH of 7.4***. Although citrus fruits in the 3.0 pH range are quite acidic, they contain only 1% the level of acids that already exist in the stomach. Thus, contrary to popular belief, they do not play a significant role in the acidity of the stomach, or in other words, *heartburn*. On the contrary, the mineral nutrients in the easy-to-digest acidic fruits and vegetables are readily absorbed, with the help of vitamin D, into the body. The acid hydrogen ions from the fruits and vegetables remain a very small part of the overall acid in the stomach. The anion nutrients (negatively charged molecules, or groups of atoms, which are attached to the positively charged hydrogen ion), such as the citrates, are all part of the *weak acid*. When these *weak acid anions* are absorbed into the body fluids, they combine with the *strong cation mineral nutrients* (positively charged molecules), such as potassium (K+) and calcium (Ca+), to form *alkali salts*, thereby lowering the acidity of the fluids in which they are contained. Therefore, *eating acidic fruits or vegetables* ***does not raise the acidity*** of the body's fluids, *but rather* ***it lowers the acidity*** of the body's fluids, *thereby helping to prevent the* ***acidosis which is the cause of disease*** (see Table 2: Food and pH).

Now that you have a better grasp of the fact that it is the lack of nutrients which causes the body fluids to become acidic resulting in disease, you will better understand just how to keep all of your body fluids alkaline and healthy. First, the most important nutrient is the sun on the skin – at least one hour each day. Also the sun must strike the pituitary gland, located behind the eyes. The next most important nutrient is the one most abundant in the human body: calcium. There are all kinds of calcium foods (see table on page 129) and there are all kinds of supplements, which are necessary to maintain adequate calcium. Calcium supplements that dissolve readily in water are the best. Try to avoid antacid calcium such as Tums®, as they destroy the precious and deficient stomach acid of the elderly, thereby inhibiting the digestion of crucial nutrients. The best form of calcium is coral calcium from Okinawa (discussed in Chapter 16, Recipes for Health). It has been consumed for 550 years and has resulted in a culture that lives to 105, disease-free with slow aging. It is becoming extremely popular all over the world, with millions of people enjoying its almost magical health benefits. Of course all other minerals and vitamins are important and will be discussed in Chapter 16, Recipes for Health.

If all of this sounds ***too simple***, that is because it basically really is simple. The scientific and medical authorities would like you to believe that, because subjects such as disease are too difficult for you to understand, you must trust them to test, measure and interpret all of the results pertaining to your health. Although this may be so for a great many things in medicine, there can be no doubt that you are, indeed, both capable of measuring, interpreting and understanding the acidity of your saliva, and thereby, the basic state of your body's fluids. These authorities think like they do because they are still suffering from the *washing-of-the-hands syndrome*, which causes them to believe that *anything too simple cannot possibly prevent disease*.

Table 2: Food and pH

Food	pH
Lemons	2.1
Vinegar	2.7
Apples	3.1
Grapefruit	3.1
Rhubarb	3.1
Strawberries	3.2
Raspberries	3.4
Tomatoes	4.2
Bananas	4.6
Carrots	5.1
Beans	5.5
Bread	5.5
Asparagus	5.6
Potatoes	5.8
Butter	6.3
Corn	6.3
Shrimp	6.9
Water	7.2
Egg Whites	7.8

CHAPTER NINE

THE BODY'S NUTRIENTS

Although these simplicities are obviously easy for you to understand, what you will find hard to understand is just how are you going to consume your seven full-course servings of fruits and vegetables that are nutritionally required to maintain good health, every day. The only realistic answer is *dietary supplements.* Also, there are additional requirements, which also must be met in order to remove the acidity of the body's fluids and maintain the required blue slightly alkaline pH of 7.4.

The first requirement, of course, is that the nutrients must be available for use by the body (see Table 3: Original Major Nutrients in the Body, and Table 4: Major Nutrients in the Blood). Our changing diets—kids drink milk and adults drink beer, and our changing lifestyles—kids play outside and adults work inside, can gradually erode our mineral nutrient stockpile to the point where the body has to rob the Peter fluid to pay the Paul fluid. There are many other, and more serious, changes, which cause mineral deficiency to occur. Much of this has been caused by the misinformation propagated by the medical establishment.

Table 3: Original Major Nutrients in the Body

Nutrient	Weight %	
* Water	39.10	* Made up of the following elements:
* Oxygen	20.30	Oxygen 65.0 %
* Glucose	19.10	Carbon 18.0 %
* Methane	13.80	Hydrogen 10.0 %
* Ammonia	2.90	Nitrogen 2.4 %
Calcium	1.60	
Iron	1.00	**Note:**
Phosphorous	0.90	The chemical breakdown of glucose
Potassium	0.40	and the chemical combination of
Sodium	0.30	oxygen with methane results in the
Chlorine	0.30	production of 34.6 % more water,
Sulfur	0.25	making a total of **73.7 % water in**
Magnesium	0.05	**the human body.**

Total 100.00

Table 4: Major Nutrients in the Blood (pH 7.3 - 7.5)

Component	Milligrams per 1000cc (ppm)*
Sodium	1400 ---1430
Chloride	1000 ---1040
Triglyceride Fat	950 ---1050
Iron	950 ---1000
Glucose	850 ---1000
LDL Cholesterol	600 ---1300
HDL Cholesterol	450 --- 850
Calcium	97 --- 106
Total Protein	72 --- 75
Potassium	40 --- 43
Phosphorus	31 --- 35

* **ppm** stands for parts per million parts of nutrients in the blood.

One example that certainly must be contrary to God's intention is the familiar medical advice, "*Stay out of the sun*," lest your skin produce the required vitamin D to allow you to absorb the required mineral nutrients, thereby preventing disease. Another myth is, "*Adults do not need to drink milk*," lest they keep their bones dense and ward off diseases like osteoporosis, arthritis, heart disease, and cancer. Besides, to get their required nutrients, the authorities could offer to let them do it the same way that the cows do it, and "*let them eat grass*." Other examples of the "*don't eat*" myths are as follows:

"**Don't eat butter,**" so that you can avoid the natural nutrients of butter while allowing the substituted margarine to provide you with enough *cis-trans fats* to dramatically increase your harmful low density cholesterol levels (LDLs).

"**Don't eat eggs,**" so that you cannot only avoid consuming cholesterol – which will later in this book be shown not to be the bad guy that it is made out to be – but by doing so, also avoid consuming *choline* which would make it difficult for your body to produce the neurotransmitter, *acetylcholine*, thereby helping to *induce senility*.

"**Don't eat extra salt,**" as too much salt causes high blood pressure. However, a recent four-year study by the prestigious Albert Einstein College of Medicine (done in association with the prestigious Cornell University Medical College) on 1,900 men with high blood pressure concluded that high blood pressure patients who ate less than five grams of salt a day had **more than four times as many heart attacks** as those who consumed over ten grams a day. Although a "**tremendous**" increase in salt can lead to a "**small**" increase in blood pressure, low sodium causes the level of renin hormone, secreted by the kidneys, in the blood to go up, and renin is found in high levels of patients with high blood pressure.

"Don't eat vitamin and mineral supplements," lest you obtain all of the nutrients that your body requires for good health. Currently, 50% of Americans consume some minerals and vitamin supplements; 25% consume them on a daily basis. A 24-year study of 11,384 people by James E. Enstrom of the University of Southern California found that taking *"vitamins and supplements cut the death rate in half."* Even more astonishing was the fact that deaths from cancers and heart disease for those taking the daily supplements was less than 10% of those who did not take the supplements. This study, by respected scientists at a prestigious institute of learning, of large numbers of people over a long time will be an excellent candidate for the AMA's wastebasket, as rather than verify the results that are crucial to the health of America, the medical establishment will demand more proof as— while Americans are dying—it withholds funding for the studies.

There is other misinformation, which does not concern food that is also propagated by the medical profession. For example: *"Your body temperature should not be allowed to rise above 98.6 degrees Fahrenheit."* What is left out of the phrase is, *"for any length of time,"* as prolonged high body temperatures can indeed cause brain damage. But, what about short periods of time, and once again, why did *God in his wisdom* make humans suffer with fevers? One answer is that many viruses and bacteria cannot survive above the body's normal temperature, and thus, the fever kills these critters. The doctor, on the other hand, is trained by the system to dispense an unnatural white chemical to quickly reduce the fever so that the virus can survive, thereby necessitating the other prescribed unnatural white chemicals known as antibiotics.

Although the doctor's method of dispensing the drug industry's expensive chemicals has succeeded in the past, there is growing evidence that it will not always continue to do so, as many virus and bacteria have begun to develop an immunity or resistance

66

to the antibiotics. But do not fret, as the drug industry is working on more unnatural antibiotics as an answer to the problem, while medicine continues to ignore *God's intended, natural way*.

Another misinformation myth is that "*Genes cause disease,*" the implication being that, because you are born with the genes that you have, there is nothing that you can do about impending disease. But not to worry, because medical research is currently spending billions of dollars working on expensive ways to give you new and healthy genes. The real tragedy with this situation is that it is the *acidosis that causes degenerative disease, and not genes.* I'm sure that you're asking, "*If this is true, then what do the genes do?*" The answer is that the *genes are the body's computer maps,* showing the body which way it can go and cannot go. Although they map the body's roadways to disease, they do not make the body go down any particular roadway. To put it in simpler terms, the genes dictate which of the many degenerative diseases to which you will be prone, they do not *cause* the disease. This concept, which is not understood by medicine today, is similar to the misconception that the sun *causes* skin cancer, when it is the *mineral deficiency-induced acidosis* which *causes the body to become prone to disease*, and the genes only pick out which one of the diseases the body will be forced to choose. For some people, their genes are programmed to choose skin cancer.

The problem with propagating this last myth that God's "*sun is bad for you*," is that just the opposite is true. The sun shining on the body's skin does many things. One result is the photosynthetic production of the mineral regulator, *inositol triphosphate* (INSP-3) an important biochemical mineral regulator. Another result of the sun shining on the skin is the photosynthesis of *vitamin D* in the skin, resulting in increasing the small intestine's capability to absorb mineral nutrients, thereby *reducing the acidosis* known to cause degenerative disease. This includes *all cancers*. As researchers know, the acid in the fluids outside and inside the human cell can disintegrate the cell wall, allowing toxins and carcinogens to get inside of the cell. Dr. James P. Whitlock Jr. of Stanford University describes carcinogens, such as dioxin, binding with receptor toxins inside of the cell to form molecules that are just the right shape and size to bind to the DNA's nucleotides. This causes the DNA template (structure) to bend or *mutate,* and *a cancer is born.*

Cancer was named by the ancients after the great veins that usually surround malignant growth; they compared these veins to the claws of a crab or "cancer" (Latin). Its origin was unknown and it was generally treated unsuccessfully with special potions and, on occasion, with local surgery.

By the turn of the twentieth century, orthodox medicine was removing growths of cancer by knife and by their destruction by *caustic applications* before glandular evolvement had supervened. At this time in history, "the use of caustics was proven to have provided a *permanent cure* in many cases" (*Health and Longetivity*, Joseph G. Richardson, M.D., University of Pennsylvania, 1909, p. 378). This procedure was usually preceded by remedies such as local bleeding and leeches, which could reduce the size of the tumor to one quarter of its original size. The *use of caustics* with potassium iodide was also used *to successfully treat rheumatism*.

"There is no disease whose prime cause is better known, so that today ignorance is no longer an excuse that one cannot do more about prevention of cancer," ("The Prime Cause and Prevention of Cancer", Otto Warburg. Lecture given by Director, Max Planck, Institute for Cell Physiology, Berlin, at the meeting of Nobel Laureates, June 30, 1966.) Warburg, two-time Nobel Prize in medicine winner, continued, *"But how long prevention will be avoided depends on how long the prophets of*

*agnosticism will succeed in **inhibiting the application of scientific knowledge in the field of cancer**. In the meantime, millions of men and women must die of cancer unnecessarily.*" (Note: in 1966 cancer struck 23% of Americans, whereas today it strikes 39% of Americans). This early work of Nobel Prize winner Otto Warburg, (**Cause and Prevention of Cancer**; *Biochem, Zeits*, 152: 514-520, 1924), showed clearly that cancer was associated with *anaerobic* (deficiency of oxygen) *conditions*, resulting in fermentation and a marked drop in the pH of the cell ("**Low pH Hyperthermia Cancer Therapy**"; *Cancer Chemotherapy Pharmacology* 4; 137-145, 1980). Moreover, the production of mutation receptors cannot occur with the ph level of the cell in the healthy calcium buffered 7.4 to 6.6 range, a range which assures the breakdown of glucose into the A, C, G and T nucleotide radicals that promote healthy DNA synthesis. M. Von Arenne showed that both high and low pH solutions *can quickly kill the cell*. He was also able to show that at a pH slightly above the normal level of 7.4, the toxic enzymes which characterize the low pH cells are neutralized, and that the cancer cells will enter a *dormant state*. Thus, the success of the "*caustic solution treatment*" of tumors by the turn-of-the-century doctors could now be explained. Also, it should be noted that by definition, alkaline solutions are made up of hydroxyl (*oxygen-hydrogen*) radicals and therefore are oxygen-rich. In the *absence of oxygen* within the acidic intracellular fluids, the *glucose undergoes fermentation into lactic acid*, causing the pH of the cell to drop even further, thereby *inhibiting the production of A, C, G and T nucleotides* that allow for normal DNA synthesis. This provides the necessary conditions for toxic enzymes to produce radicals that will bond with carcinogens. The complexes they produce will bind with specific sequences of nucleotides in the DNA, causing the template to be altered, thereby setting the scene for the abnormal replication of DNA to trigger cancer.

It should be understood that the connection of acidosis to cancer has been well-defined by medical researchers, and the fact that cancers do not do well when the acid is removed, is well understood by today's cancer researchers. In fact, one of the leading cancer researchers in America, when asked by a significant cancer research contributor—a friend of mine who had seen his prostate cancer disappear after taking vitamins and mineral supplements to reduce his acidosis and raise his body fluid pH—explained that, "*Of course, everyone knows that cancer cannot survive in an alkali.*" When then asked the obvious question, "*Then why don't you just make the body alkaline?*" he responded, "*We just don't know how to do this.*" Of course the "**we**" refers to orthodox medicine, which has little to no training in nutrition.

Another friend of mine, a retired high-ranking naval veteran, claimed that his progressing skin cancer—diagnosed by doctors—had been caused by chemicals used in the Vietnam War. He was told that except for repetitive surgery, nothing could be done. However, after raising his saliva pH from yellow 5.0 to blue 7.5 by taking thirty cents per day worth of vitamins and minerals daily, and by taking lots of sunshine for four months, and by maintaining his saliva at a pH of 7.5 for one year at a cost of fifteen cents per day, no trace of skin cancer remained. Caustic body fluids had killed the cancer, much like the caustic applications of the turn-of-the-century doctors had done. The maintenance of caustic body fluids was aided by the sunshine-produced vitamin D. Although exposure to sunshine by cancer victims is deplored by orthodox medicine, the father of medicine, Dr. Hippocrates, endorsed it.

Thus, the question of whether God's sunshine is good for your health is obviously so important that it should not be the responsibility of those making the claim that *the sun is good for your health* to prove the correctness of their claim to the governing medical authorities. Already massive scientific literature is available supporting the importance of sunshine to health. This literature concludes that high serum calcium levels are a direct result of decalcification of the bones for the purpose of supplying calcium to the organs which are desperate for calcium. It is also due to a lack of sunshine, resulting in low calcium-regulating calcitonin production and calcium-storage inisotol triphosphate production. Calcium deficiency due to lack of calcium in the diet, along with lack of exposure to sunshine, are responsible for hypercalcemia. Vitamin D, produced by sunshine, allows the body to absorb large quantities of calcium and therefore helps to prevent hypercalcemia. Also, the sunshine that produces vitamin D also causes the pituitary gland to instruct the parathyroid gland to produce the hormone, calcitonin, which prevents the decalcification of the bones. Thus, vitamin D *actually prevents the health problems that it is accused of causing.*

When the vitamin D receptors (VDRs) in the small intestine are saturated with vitamin D, the body can increase its absorption of calcium 20-fold, thereby minimizing allergy. The sun is the best source of vitamin D. In an article by P.C. Beadle entitled, **"Cholecalciferol Production,"** Beadle describes how he measured the vitamin D production in the epidermis (skin) to be 163 IUs per square centimeter in light skin per day and 69 IUs per square centimeter in dark skin per day. As the human body has 20 square feet of skin (18,580 square centimeters) the daily production of vitamin D is between 1,000,000 and 3,000,000 IUs, demonstrating that the Recommended Daily Allowance (RDA) of 400 IUs could be produced within 6 to 18 seconds of sunshine. This proves that the RDA for vitamin D is ludicrously low. Evidence points to a prostrate, breast and colon cancer belt in the United States which lies in the northern latitudes. Rates for these cancers are two to three times higher than in the sunnier South. Thus, allergy is also less prevalent in the South.

And finally, a 1997 study by the North California Cancer Center concluded that, *"because the skin uses ultraviolet rays from the sun to make vitamin D* [which has been linked to protection against breast cancer in other studies which confirmed

71

that woman from states in the tier south of Kansas tend to get significantly less breast cancer], that the *risk of breast cancer is lowered by 40%, perhaps even more, by exposure to sunlight.*"

The financial burden of further proof that sunshine is beneficial to health should be borne by the establishment. In fact, if it is truly protecting the health of America, it should be responsible for financing the *third-party research* to either prove or to disprove any medical claim. The assessment of the results should also be made by a *third-party group* that does not have the same *prejudice that burdens the current establishment*, which is not only judge and jury, but also lavishes in the responsibility of being the *prosecutor*, or, in other words, "*three strikes and your out and the balls have already been thrown.*" They take this position despite all of the current massive scientific evidence that disputes their position.

For the sake of human health, the burden of proof should be shifted to the well-funded establishment. The onus should be on the establishment to prove, right or wrong, any claims made. For failure to do so results in the suppression of legitimate medical advancements at a cost of great human suffering. The stakes are too high to allow the AMA and the FDA to hide behind their feeble pass-the-buck response of, *"the burden of proof is on those making the claim."* History has shown that scientific proof that does not conform to the establishment's preconceived concepts is always rejected initially; just ask Nobel Prize winners Max Planck, Albert Einstein, and Linus Pauling.

Unfortunately, the current establishment is burdened with the *unwarranted fear* that, by proving the correctness of the claim that *degenerative disease could be cured by eliminating acidosis,* they may also be *eliminating doctors' jobs.* This misconception will be discussed in more detail in the last chapter.

CHAPTER TEN

THE HUMAN CELL

Now that the reader is familiar with the concept that degenerative disease thrives in acidic body fluids and that the same *disease cannot survive in an alkaline fluid*, it is time to try to attempt to explain some of the many reasons.

To begin with, one basic quality that *alkaline fluids* have over acidic fluids is their *ability to absorb gases*. For example, some alkaline fluids have many times more capacity to absorb oxygen than acidic fluids. Thus, the oxygen-rich, alkaline body fluids are more capable of *killing a virus* than the oxygen poor, acidic, body fluids. Also, humans are creatures requiring lots of oxygen for numerous biological functions, therefore, alkaline fluids are more conducive to biological functions than acidic fluids.

The question therefore becomes, "*Why do biological functions prefer alkaline fluids?*" Once again, oxygen is largely responsible, as alkalis are hydroxides by definition and hydroxides are composed of oxygen and hydrogen (see Table 1: pH). The surface membrane of each cell is composed of a *bilayer of phospholipids,* which could be compared to an air mattress composed of two layers of balloons, with the upper and lower layers bound together by string. The phospholipid layers are largely bound together by that unwanted chemical known as *cholesterol.* The surface of the phospholipid balloons contains significant oxygen, which makes it **hydrophilic**, or, in other words, water and fluids are attracted to it. This cloud of oxygen also makes it very **negatively charged**, thereby allowing the surface to capture cancer-causing chemicals, most of which are made up of derivatives of the electron-starved benzene. These positively charged carcinogens stick to the negatively charged surface, and, like flies to flypaper, are eliminated from any activity. The cell surface can hold a lifetime of these pesky critters, within reasonable limits, but unlike the flypaper that holds the flies until they die, the cell only holds the carcinogens until the cell dies and disintegrates. Once liberated, the carcinogen can get inside the ruptured cell, where it **induces cell mutation**.

T he oxygen-rich, negatively charged cell surface also attracts the positively charged minerals, such as calcium and magnesium, which then attract negative nutrients in preparation for entry into the cell. The nutrients enter the cell through a **nutrient channel** which is kept closed by a rosette of coiled proteins, like a coiled snake plugging a hole, bound together by calcium. When the rosette snake uncoils, it makes an opening, which allows the mineral stacked nutrients to enter the cell. The rosette of proteins coils or stretches as required because of changing chemical charges. The difference between the slightly acidic pH of the fluid inside the cell – which continues to drop as the nutrients inside are consumed in biochemical reactions – and the constantly high pH 7.4, of the fluids outside the cell, generates an electrical potential difference (an electrical voltage). When the charge becomes large enough, it causes the positively charged end of the rosette snake coil to stretch towards the negatively charged external fluids, thereby opening the cell and allowing the higher pH nutrients to flow through the nutrient channel into the cell. These high pH fluids entering the cell in turn raise the pH inside the cell, thereby lowering the electrical charge, allowing the rosette snake to recoil and plug the channel.

Thus, the cell has been opened and closed electrically. Therefore, electrophysiology is a reality, despite the numerous condemnations from the medical establishment. One can easily imagine an external electrical charge superimposing its negative voltage on the cell, causing it to remain open. The result would be biological havoc. Of course, both the medical authorities and the utility companies would have difficulty envisioning such spooks.

When the main nutrient, which is the *sugar glucose*, enters the cell, it begins to undergo immediate changes that are dependent on the pH or degree of acidity inside the cell. For example, if the inner cell fluids are at a pH of 6.0 or lower, the acid causes the six carbon glucose to split in half, forming two lactic acid molecules (each containing three carbons), which thereby drops the pH even further. This acid results in cell-surface disintegration, which liberates the carcinogens and toxins for entry into the ruptured cell. If, on the other hand, the fluids inside the cell are at the more alkaline pH of 6.5 or higher, only one or two of the carbons are removed from the 6 carbon glucose. This can allow the four nucleotides containing four and five carbons – which are the basic building blocks of DNA – to be formed. Thus, in an acidic environment, the *DNA, which is Mother Nature's blueprint for the body* cannot be formed. This is probably the main reason why acidosis results in degenerative diseases, and why raising the body fluid's pH can result in curing the disease.

This brings up the question of aging. If, as described in the previous paragraph, acidosis prevents the formation of nucleotides, which are the building blocks of DNA, which is the blueprint for human growth, then how can an acidic body grow and repair itself? In other words, acidosis slows down growth and body repair, which are two of the basic traits of aging. This is probably why people who are very sick with disease look very old, and when health returns, they regain some youth. What this means to the layperson is that there really may be *a fountain of youth,* and it would be in the form of *alkaline body fluids.*

Archeologists studying the cultures of the past 700,000 years have discovered that those who lived in hunting cultures had strong bones and were slim and relatively disease-free, while those from agricultural cultures (starting 10,000 years ago) had weak bones, cavities and were disease-prone. Diet was therefore the key factor. Agricultural cultures began consuming large amounts of carbohydrates, which are readily converted to glucose. The pancreas must then produce large quantities of insulin to convert the glucose into collagen and fat. The high insulin also causes the body to produce cholesterol necessary to construct new cells to store the fat. The result is high blood pressure, high cholesterol, acidosis from the sugar, and fat storage. The hunting cultures are eating a high-protein, low-carbohydrate diet, resulting in low glucose. This causes the pancreas to produce glucagon, which removes the fat from the cells to produce fuel for the body. The health hunter's original protein to carbohydrate (*procarb*) ratio was **1 to 1**. In America today, pastas, pizzas and pies raise the procarb ratio to about **1 to 4**. Biologically, 10,000 generations are required to adjust to a major change in diet, but the human body has only had 500 generations to adjust to about a **1 to 2** procarb ratio. The human body is therefore currently not designed for a **1 to 4** procarb diet.

Another aspect of the human cell that should be taught to the layperson is the fact that the nutrient channel is a one-way mechanism. Fluids and nutrients can only enter the cell through the channel and cannot leave through the same opening. There are, however, smaller channels that allow both fluids and some

76

small minerals, such as sodium and the similar-sized calcium, to exit the cell. This is an important phenomenon, as it has *allowed some researchers* and some cultures around the world *to defeat disease*, even the dreaded cancer. Dr. Max Gerson of New York City was famous for curing the incurables of the world, the most famous being Albert Schweitzer. Dr. Gerson had noted that his cancer patients had an abnormally high amount of the mineral potassium in their blood. Gerson reasoned that as the potassium ions (dissolved potassium mineral), which were twice as big as the sodium and calcium ions, could never make it out of the cell through the smaller sodium or calcium channels, the cell membrane surface must have ruptured. Believing that the cells would therefore need more of this required nutrient in order to repair themselves, Dr. Gerson—to the absolute horror of his medical colleagues—began giving his cancer patients a mixture of three potassium salts: potassium glauconate, potassium acetate and potassium phosphate. The result, an astounding success for the patients, brought the standard reply of, *"quackery"* from the establishment. The strongly alkaline potassium had raised the pH of the inner cell fluids, thereby killing the acid-loving cancer. All this was done without the pain and side effects of chemotherapy or radiation. As the therapy was also inexpensive, Dr. Gerson became a pre-convicted medical maverick.

Cancer is virtually unknown to the Hunza population in Northern Pakistan. Remember that one in three Americans will contract cancer, and the rate of cancer deaths has increased by over 50% in just the past 20 years (see Table 5: U.S. Cancer Deaths). Their water is both rich in potassium and in *cesium, potassium's bigger cousin*. Cesium, in fact, is the most caustic mineral known, and it is able to just barely make it into the cell through the nutrient channel. Once inside, it can never leave, thereby assuring that the fluids inside of the cell remain caustic. Thus, cancer can never take hold. Because the cesium is found in the water, it is also consumed by the plants, which are eaten by the locals, further ensuring a cancer-free environment. Medical authorities in America have responded by preventing the public from purchasing this supposedly *"potentially dangerous"* mineral, that is very effective at quickly reversing acidosis.

Table 5: U.S. Cancer Deaths

Year	Deaths
1970	329,000
1975	365,000
1978	405,000
1985	462,000
1990	514,000

Source: American Cancer Society

Another culture that is almost cancer-free is the Hopi Indian band in northern Arizona. They are surrounded by an ocean of cancer, but on their reservation they are protected by their water which contains the mineral *rubidium*, potassium's bigger cousin and cesium's smaller cousin. It is also very caustic, and when inside of the cell, quickly eliminates both the acid and the cancer.

To the average American, these facts may seem incredulous. How could a cure for cancer exist without the whole world knowing about it? That is a question that should be answered by the medical authorities. They should be forced to use facts and not be allowed to use their accustomed name-calling rhetoric. Even in America, as far back as 1909, Joseph G. Richardson, in his book *Health and Longevity*, describes *"the removal of cancerous growths by the knife or their destruction by caustic applications"* (page 378). In 1924, a medical researcher, Dr. Otto Warburg, wrote in his book *Cause and Prevention of Cancer* (pages 514-520) that with cancerous cells, the *"oxygen deficiency induces fermentation which results in a marked drop in the pH of the cell.* Sound familiar? Of course, despite the fact that his work was totally ignored by the medical authorities, in 1932, Dr. Warburg won the Nobel Prize for demonstrating that cancer was anaerobic (lives in an environment without oxygen). Unfortunately, as was the case with all the other Nobel Prize winners, Dr. Warburg spent the rest of his life fighting the governing establishment.

In 1979, Dr. K. Brewer described in a publication, *The Mechanisms of Carcinogenesis* (*Journal of IAPM*, Volume V, No. 2) the use of cesium and rubidium salt to treat cancer patients. In 1985, Dr. H. Sartori described in a publication, *Cancer, Orwellian or Eutopian?* (Life Science Universal Inc.), the successful treatment of terminal cancer patients with cesium salts. In the latter study, initiated in April 1981, fifty terminal cancer patients with only days to live, and three of whom were comatose, were given vitamins, minerals and *cesium chloride.* Ten of the patients had breast cancer; nine had colon cancer; six had prostrate cancer; four had pancreas cancer; five had lung cancer; three had liver cancer; three had lymphoma; one had Ewing sarcoma pelvis; one had adeno cancer; and eight had unknown primary cancer. With all fifty patients, conventional treatment had failed and the patients had been sent home to die. The chances of even one surviving were one in a million. Amazingly, after two weeks of cesium treatment, only twelve had died (including all three comatose patients), and their autopsies showed that their cancer was benign at the time of death. The cesium treatment was continued for two more weeks and after one year *the survival rate was an incredible 50 %.* Further research was carried out jointly by Brewer and Sartori with even greater success. Both men have been persecuted, ridiculed and belittled by the medical establishment, for whom the results of their work remains totally ignored to this day, while cesium is now forbidden.

There are also dozens of recent studies by credible research facilities demonstrating the fact that cancer can be prevented through nutrition. For example, a 25-year study ending in 1997 by the Finland National Public Health Institute on 4,697 cancer-free women aged 15 to 90, concluded that there was *"an overwhelming association between the high consumption of milk and the prevention of breast cancer compared to other factors."* Also, a 1997 study by the Northern California Cancer Center concluded that, "because the skin uses ultraviolet rays from the sun to make vitamin D (which has been linked to protection against breast cancer in other studies which confirmed that woman from states in the tier south of Kansas tend to get significantly less breast cancer), that the *risk of breast cancer is lowered by 40%, perhaps even more by exposure to sunlight."*Another 1997 study published in the *Journal of the National Cancer Institute,* by UCLA's Johnson Cancer Center showed that by putting American women on a diet that mimics foods—including fish oil rich in vitamin D—eaten by Asian women, who have a much lower rate of breast cancer than American women, increased omega-3 fatty acid levels in the women (omega-3 suppresses tumor growth in mice and in cultures) to the level of the Asian women, and in only three months. However, in true American fashion and probably out of fear of offending the drug industry, the study *"cautioned"* that the research *"does not prove* that a diet rich in fish oil would prevent breast cancer." Intriguingly, when Asian women come to America and adopt the low-fish-oil diet of Americans, their rate of breast cancer skyrockets. Thus, the highly regulated American medical research industry is afraid to admit the truth. Instead, they imply that it *"may be true,"* and you should continue taking drugs while they continue their research into the matter. Unfortunately, the victims with breast cancer are the ones who pay the price for this incredible indifference to scientific facts by the medical community.

The story is almost always the same: The medical work was successful; the researchers either won prestigious awards before being ostracized by the authorities, who belittled their work, or the researchers waffled on their conclusions out of fear of offending the establishment. Either way, the result is the maintenance of a state of ignorance by the public regarding the medical capability to defeat disease. This is maintained despite the numerous scientific publications loaded with powerful evidence that "disease can be prevented through nutrition."

Another example is biochemist, Dr. Anghiler, who in 1985 stated in the book, *The Role of Calcium in Biological Systems*, that, *"It can be demonstrated that many of the unorthodox cancer treatments may indeed have scientific merit, and, **when chemically understood, cancer may be beaten painlessly.**" Wow!!!*

By the late 1990s, other medical men of wisdom were also discovering that calcium supplements could indeed reverse cancer. In the October 13, 1998 issue of the *New York Times* an article appeared entitled, *"Calcium Takes Its Place As a Superstar of Nutrients"* in which it reports that a study published in the *Journal of the American Medical Association* reported that "increasing calcium induced normal development of the epithelia cells and might also prevent cancer in such organs as the breast, prostate and pancreas." It also reported that the *American Journal of Clinical Nutrition* published "virtually no major organ system escapes calcium's influence" and that a research team from the University of Southern California found "adding calcium to the diet lowered the blood pressure in 110 black teenagers."

The January 14, 1999 issue of the *Phoenix Republic* wrote in an article entitled *"Calcium Reduces Tumors"* that the *New England Journal of Medicine* reported "adding calcium to the diet can keep you from getting tumors in your large intestine." Then the February 1999 issue of *Reader's Digest* wrote in an article entitled, *"The 'Superstar' Nutrient"* that the *Journal of the*

American Medical Association published, "When the participants' consumption reached 1,500 milligrams of calcium a day, cell growth in the colon improved toward normal (this means that the cancer was reversed)." The *Digest* also reported that the Metabolic Bone Center at St. Luke's Hospital believes that "a chronic deficiency of calcium is largely responsible for premenstrual syndrome (PMS)" and that "a lot of women are avoiding the sun and their vitamin D levels may be very low." In the same article, the *Digest* reported, "in 1997, the large, federally financed trial found that a diet containing 1,200 milligrams of calcium significantly lowered blood pressure in adults." Then the May 3, 1999 edition of *US World News Report* wrote in an article entitled, *"Calcium's Powerful Mysterious Ways,"* that "Researchers are increasingly finding that the humble mineral calcium plays a major role in warding off major illnesses from high blood pressure to colon cancer" and that "You name the disease, and calcium is beginning to have a place there" (David McCarron, nephrologist at Oregon Health Sciences University). Unfortunately, most doctors have not heard the news that their own journals, major, popular newspapers and magazines are reporting that natural supplements, especially calcium, can cure and prevent disease.

CHAPTER ELEVEN

CHOLESTEROL

Now that the reader has become familiar with the body's fluids and the human cell, it is time to clear up another popular misconception: "*Cholesterol is bad for you*." Actually, no one ever really tells you that cholesterol is bad for you. However, what they do say is that *a high cholesterol level in your blood can kill you*. It is this threat of death that leaves the reader with the implication that cholesterol must be bad for you. This is simply not the case.

To begin with, cholesterol should be defined. Cholesterol is defined as a secondary alcohol. Compared to the alcohol in the spirits we consume, the two-carbon ethanol, cholesterol is a giant molecule with 27 carbons. It is a cousin to one form of vitamin D, cholecalciferol, that also has 27 carbons. It is found in large amounts of unsaturated fatty acids and eggs (one egg contains about 300 milligrams of cholesterol). The body produces about 2,000 mg of cholesterol each day, and that is why studies have shown that when most cholesterol is removed from the diet, the cholesterol level in the blood remains basically the same. This is not to say that a diet rich in cholesterol will not raise your blood cholesterol, because usually it will. Cholesterol is like any other nutrient in that too much of anything is probably not good for your health. For example, too much sugar or too much salt can kill you, and yet the public hysteria has been directed at the bad guy, cholesterol. To a biochemist, this situation is ridiculous, as cholesterol is one of the more predominant molecules in the human body. It binds and holds the bilayer cell walls together. It is the base chemical from which many hormones are derived, including testosterone and estrogen (sex hormones). It is used to conduct nerve impulses. It is present in large quantities in the brain and bile. *Cholesterol is a necessity for life.*

Cholesterol combines with various fatty acids in the blood to form two types of protein salts known as lipoproteins. One type is known as high-density lipoprotein, or *HDL cholesterol — known as the good cholesterol*, as people who have high levels of it in their blood actually have less risk of heart disease. The other type is known as low-density lipoprotein — or *LDL cholesterol — known as the bad cholesterol*, as people who have high levels of it in their blood are prone to heart disease.

As was discussed previously, becoming prone to heart disease does not mean that the LDL cholesterol *causes the heart disease*, but rather, it makes the body more prone to getting heart disease in lieu of getting other degenerative diseases. It is not only an oversimplification to state that because cholesterol is found in significant amounts in the arterial plaque, blocking the flow of blood, that cholesterol is responsible and therefore should be avoided. In fact, this is simply not true. If society were to use the same deductive reasoning, we would have to throw all policemen in jail because – just like cholesterol – they are always found at the scene of the crime. Ironically, both police and cholesterol are at the crime scene for the same reason: *they are there to help save your life.*

To understand the role of cholesterol in plaque buildup, it is first necessary to ask yourself the following question: *"If cholesterol in my blood is so bad for me, then why don't I ever develop plaque in my veins?"* After all, it is the same blood, in the same heart, in the same body. This question should be addressed to your doctor. The answer lies in the basic difference between a blood artery and a blood vein. The artery, which delivers blood from the heart to various parts of the body, is basically the same as a vein, which returns the blood to the heart, but with one major difference: The artery surface is made up of muscle tissue that can squeeze and compress the artery, resulting in an increased blood pressure, thereby ensuring blood gets to the distant parts of the body. It is muscle tissue that is most susceptible to disintegration by lactic acid. Once the body's fluids become acidic, the muscle-tissue surface of the arteries becomes a susceptible target. The April 1997 issue of the *New England Journal of Medicine* agrees with this concept by suggesting a radical *"new"* medical theory that cholesterol is not the primary *"cause"* of heart disease, but rather, *"inflammation of blood vessel walls is the primary cause of heart attacks and strokes."* With the muscle tissue disintegrated, the remainder of the artery wall is weakened. Should the artery break, death would be certain. To prevent this from happening, the body responds by reinforcing the weakened arterial wall. As the wall is thin, it is exposed to the very *positively charged* external acids (acids are positively charged and alkalis are negative). This causes various components in the blood with *negatively charged components*, such as phospholipids, to be attracted and stick to the positive, acid-weakened wall. A host of other components – collagen, triglycerides, fibrin, mucopolysaccarides, heavy metals, proteins, muscle tissue and debris, and *finally,* the crack-sealing, goopy LDL cholesterol, can now attach themselves to the phospholipids anchored on the weakened artery wall. All of these plaque components are bound together by calcium.

The net result is a stronger, but thickened and hardened, artery wall, which diminishes the size of the opening in the artery.

This plaque-filled state of the arteries is known as *heart disease*. It was *caused by acidosis,* which was the result of *mineral deficiency.* Cholesterol, along with nine other components in the blood, worked together to prevent a break in the artery that would have resulted in rapid death. It is, therefore, true that the more cholesterol there is in the blood, the easier it becomes for it to do its job of *saving the life of the body.* Unfortunately, cholesterol was found at the scene of the crime, and it has been *judged guilty* by medical justice.

M edicine first approaches the problem of plaque buildup by prescribing cholesterol-lowering drugs. These statin and fibrate drugs, such as Lovastatin marketed as Mevacor® and Gemfibrozil marketed as Lopid®, do indeed work to lower the blood cholesterol levels and are therefore very popular with the pill pushers and make billions of dollars for the drug industry. In fact, in the past decade, prescriptions of drugs to lower cholesterol and other fats have increased tenfold. In 1992 alone, 26 million U.S. prescriptions were filled by doctors. As all drugs can have major and minor side effects, a review of the Lovastatin and Gemfibrozil side effects is warranted. The *Consumer Guide of Prescription Drugs* lists the possible *side effects of Mevacor*® as follows: abdominal pain, altered sense of taste, constipation, cramps, diarrhea, dizziness, flatulence, headache, heartburn, itching, nausea, rash, stomach upset, blurred vision, clouding of the eyes, difficulty swallowing, fever, liver disorders, malaise, muscle aches, and tingling of the fingers and toes. The list of the possible *side effects of Lopid*® is as follows: abdominal pain, change in taste, constipation, diarrhea, dizziness, fatigue, headache, muscle pain, nausea, stomach upset, chills, dark urine, fever, irregular heartbeat, skin rash, sore throat, vomiting, yellowing of the eyes or skin, and numbness or tingling of hands or feet. To top it off, researchers have now discovered that cholesterol-lowering drugs cause cancer in mice and rats. Studies have found that Lovastatin, when administered at blood concentrations just two to four times the levels seen in the

maximum doses that might be prescribed to patients, caused a higher than normal incidence of stomach, liver, and lung tumors in mice. At somewhat higher levels, other statin drugs caused rodent cancers. Of course the drug industry will argue that drugs that cause cancer in rodents ***may not do so in humans***, but it is your life with which they are gambling.

When the cholesterol-lowering drugs fail, then medicine approaches the problem by using a very expensive scalpel to surgically remove and replace the damaged section of the artery. The only problem with this is that they did not remove the cause— acid fluids dissolving the arterial muscle tissue—and thus the problem reoccurs to the point where surgery is necessary, on average, every four years. Also, this surgery is not without risk, as ten percent die. One heart surgeon told me that one day after having done a lifetime of thousands of triple and quadruple bypasses, he saw the scarred chest of a veteran patient on his operating table. Although he knew the patient well, he was taken aback by the obvious signs of several surgeries on the patient's chest. He thought to himself, "*What am I doing? This is assembly-line surgery that only sets the disease back temporarily. This is the fourth time that this poor guy has been on my table.*" The patient died during surgery. Seeing the doctor in despair, one nurse gave comfort to him by explaining that there was a way that he could truly help his patients. It was called ***chelation therapy***. After sadly recanting this story to me he then proudly continued, "*Since that day I have successfully treated over two thousand heart patients with chelation therapy, and I have not lost one yet. And to top it off, my patients are generally cured of heart disease. Oh sure there are some problems. For example, they only spend $2,000 on chelation therapy, when they could have been spending $50,000 on a bypass. I am not making quite as much money as I used to, but I sure feel good about myself.*"

So, what is chelation therapy, and why doesn't my doctor recommend it? The "why" is partly answered by the last part of the previous quote. The first part of the question, "what is it?"

can be readily explained to the layperson. The word "*chelation*" comes from the Greek word "*chela*," which means crab, as a crab has many claws with which to grab many things at the same time. In the case of chelation therapy, the chelating agent is a natural substance extracted from plants known as **EDTA (or ethylene diamine tetraacetic acid** for those of us who love chemistry). This natural acid loves to dissolve and grab up the calcium in the arterial plaque, which then disintegrates. Chelation therapy is done both carefully and slowly over time so as not to liberate too much plaque residue at any one time, thereby reducing the risk of a brain embolism. It is usually given by a series of injections into the blood under a doctor's supervision. Most major American cities have at least one chelation clinic.

The interesting question then becomes, "*Who discovered chelation therapy and when was it first used?*" Although several people have claimed credit, the real use was probably over one thousand years ago. Many cultures have used plants and herbs for thousands of years to treat heart disease, with many claims of success. It remains to be seen whether these plants contain a natural chelating agent. More recently – as one story goes – while treating toxic metal poisoning with a bitter tea made from desert plants, the Indians ended up curing one doctor's heart disease. Having analyzed the chemistry of the tea concoction, the doctor believed the active component that removed arterial plaque to be sodium EDTA. The rest is history, or so the story goes. This story may actually have some merit, as EDTA has been used for years by the oil industry to remove **cement plaque**, by dissolving the calcium compounds from damaged well bores (the author has personal experience chelating wells). Thus, Western science is well aware of EDTA's chelating capabilities, and if found in the Indian tea, would recognize how their medicine actually works.

The bottom line on chelation therapy is that it works to *dissolve and remove the plaque in all of the body's arteries.*

However, unless the cause of the plaque, acidosis, is resolved by nutritional therapy, the plaque will return. The therapist may also recommend that chelation therapy not be used if there is concern that the breakup of massive plaque could lead to an embolism. If this is the case, and even if it is not the case, *nutritional therapy should be instituted* in order to balance the body's nutrients. This results in the gradual dissolution of plaque.

At this point, it is time to stress the fact that nutritional therapy is not *what the doctor ordered.* A trained nutritionist is recommended. Chapter 16, Recipes For Health, will also provide some guidance. One must not try to avoid cholesterol, for by doing so, necessary nutritious food, such as eggs, are left out of the diet, and substitutes, such as margarine instead of butter, do more harm than good. An example of this last case is the research that found that eating a diet of partially hydrogenated fats, or trans fats (margarine), increased the bad LDL cholesterol level in the blood, while reducing the good HDL level (Ronald P. Mensink, Martin B. Katan, *New England Journal of Medicine*, August 1990). Nutritionist Dr. Margaret A. Flynn at the University of Missouri, found in a carefully controlled experiment involving 71 faculty members that, "Basically, it made no difference to the blood cholesterol level whether they ate margarine or butter." This is because, although butter adds cholesterol to the body, margarine's trans fats induce the body to produce more cholesterol. Nutritionists and biochemists have known for years that the *doctor's advice to his elderly patients to switch from butter to margarine is absolutely wrong*.

In fact, scientists have been lobbying governments for years to put warning labels on margarine. Biochemist Dr. Bruce J. Holub at the University of Guelph in Canada states, "*At the very least, one has to ask whether cholesterol -free claims should be allowed on high trans fat products such as margarine.*" Other researchers found that feeding animals *pure cholesterol does not lead to heart disease*, unless the cholesterol is heat damaged or oxidized. For example, a boiled egg has less LDL cholesterol than a fried egg. In the *Encyclopedia of Biochemistry*, Dr. W. Hartroft states, *"It has still not been shown that lowering the cholesterol in the blood (by 20%) will have any protective effect for the heart and vessels against the development of atheroma (hardening of the arteries), and the onset of serious complications."* Since Dr. Hartcroft made this statement, there have been many carefully controlled experiments carried out that have confirmed that *low cholesterol diets do not reduce heart disease.*

One interesting study that did show a reduction in heart disease was done by the British Medical Research Council. It was a 10-year study that looked at the health of 5,000 men aged 45 to 59 at the start of the study. Scientists monitored heart disease along with several other factors, including diet. They were astounded by the results that prove a definite link to milk reducing the incidence of heart disease. Only 1% of those who drank more than one half-liter of milk each day suffered heart attacks in the study period, against 10% of those who drank no milk at all (*a tenfold difference*). Also, drinking more than one half-liter of milk each day further reduced the incidence of heart disease. Dr. Ann Fehely, one of the team's researchers concluded that, *"The association between milk-drinking and lowered heart attack risk is clear, and there was no significance about what type of milk—full, semi-skimmed or full-skimmed—as the key ingredient was calcium."* The essential ingredients that do not change with the skimming of milk are the mineral nutrients, *especially calcium*.

Also, as was noted in the previous chapter, the 25-year study ending in 1997 by the Finland National Public Health Institute on 4,697 cancer-free women aged 15 to 90, concluded that there was *"an overwhelming association between the high consumption of milk and the prevention of breast cancer compared to other factors."*

Another recent study done on 459 people by the National Institutes for Health reported in the April 1997 issue of the *New England Journal of Medicine* concluded that "*a diet rich in fruits and vegetables and low fat dairy products can reduce blood pressure* as much as the most commonly used hypertension drugs, eliminating the need for expensive drugs for many patients with hypertension." It further went on to say, "the study was not designed to identify which components of the diet were responsible for its beneficial effects, but experts speculate that *the calcium in milk may confer the greatest blood pressure-lowering benefits*." The study also stated "widespread adoption of the combination diet could *reduce the risk of heart disease by 15 percent* and the likelihood of *stroke by 27 percent*. Dr. George Blackburn, president of the American Society for Clinical Nutrition, stated, "with nearly 50 million Americans having hypertension, and considering the billions of dollars spent each year on blood pressure medications, these findings have important public-health considerations."

Also of note was another 24-year study, ending in 1996, of 11,384 people by James E. Enstrom of the University of Southern California that found that taking *vitamins and supplements cut the death rate in half*. Even more astonishing was the fact that *deaths from cancers and heart disease* for those taking the daily supplements *were less than 10% of those who did not take the supplements*. This study, by respected scientists at a prestigious institute of learning, of large numbers of people over a long time will be an excellent candidate for the AMA's wastebasket, as rather than verify the results that are crucial to the health of America, the medical establishment will demand more proof as, while Americans are dying, it withholds funding for the studies.

What makes all of these studies tragic is that they meet all of the prerequisites for scientific authentication that is apparently required by the AMA, and yet all these studies go unheeded, despite the fact that they could potentially *reduce the death rate of both heart disease and cancer, the number one and two killers in America, by "tenfold" while also reducing strokes by 27%*, as well as providing a means for women to prevent the dreaded breast cancer, thereby preventing massive human suffering while saving millions of lives. The fortunate drug companies – and the doctors of America – reap hundreds of billions of dollars per year because of this AMA *indifference to using milk nutrition to prevent heart disease and caustic nutrition to prevent cancer*. This indifference is also paid for with human suffering as well as hundreds of thousands of lives each year.

The medical authorities claim to need proof for claims regarding benefits to health. The previously mentioned studies were long, massive, and done at a very prestigious scientific establishment by world-renowned scientists. None of these scientists have yet won a Nobel Prize, so that cannot be used against them. As the rate of occurrence of all degenerative diseases in America is currently rising at almost epidemic proportions, the *war on disease is definitely not being won; it is definitely being lost!* You would think that it would be logical for the American medical establishment to eagerly adopt such *massive studies which potentially show a means of reducing heart disease and cancer by as much as tenfold while reducing strokes by 27% and dramatically reducing breast cancer in women*. An added incentive should be the fact that the father of medicine, Hippocrates, taught 2,500 years ago that *the best food is the best medicine*, and since very few in science would dispute that *milk, fruits, and vegetables are some of the best foods* – as has been demonstrated by these massive studies – the doctors should leap at the chance to not only practice the Hippocratic code of ethics, but to also practice the preventive medicine which Hippocrates believed in and practiced. Unfortunately, the modern development of food supplements was not available to Hippocrates who, because of their food source, would most assuredly have endorsed their use.

CHAPTER TWELVE

THE CALCIUM FACTOR

The reader, by now, has become familiar with some of the basic concepts in biochemistry that are pertinent to human health. Up to now, although the critical importance of mineral nutrients has been explained, no one mineral nutrient has yet been suggested as being more important than the others. Of course, every mineral nutrient is necessary to sustain life, as we know it. However, there are some minerals, which have several more biological functions than others, and therefore, a deficiency of these minerals in the body causes many more biological problems (human ailments) than those with fewer functions. The mineral nutrient with the most biological functions is calcium.

Calcium, a metallic element that makes up 3.4 % of the earth's crust, the fifth most abundant element (see Table 6: *Elemental Composition of the Earth's Crust Versus the Human Body*), was not identified as an element until the early nineteenth century. It was named after the lime, *calk*, which the Romans first prepared in the first century. It is never found in nature uncombined and occurs abundantly in the carbonate form as limestone. *Calcium is also the **most abundant** mineral nutrient (1.6 % by weight) in the human body.*

TABLE 6: ELEMENTAL COMPOSITION OF THE EARTH'S CRUST VERSUS THE HUMAN BODY

Element	% Earth's Crust	% Human Body
Oxygen	49.00	65.00
Silicon	26.00	trace
Aluminum	7.50	trace
Iron	4.70	1.00
Calcium	**3.40**	**1.60**
Sodium	2.60	0.30
Potassium	2.40	0.40
Magnesium	1.90	0.05
Hydrogen	0.88	10.00
Titanium	0.55	trace
Chlorine	0.19	0.30
Phosphorus	0.12	0.90
Carbon	0.09	18.0
Manganese	0.08	0.00
Sulfur	0.03	0.25
Nitrogen	0.02	2.40
Total	**99.46**	**100.00**

Note: All other non-manmade elements (77 elements) make up 0.54 % of the earth's crust.

It should be noted that carbon, one of the elements lowest in concentration in the earth's crust, is one of the elements highest in concentration in the human body. But, carbon is basically only a structural component of the body, and must be combined with one or more elements, such as hydrogen, in molecular form to be functionally active. This compounding renders both the carbon and the hydrogen much less reactive than calcium, which is, therefore, much more capable of diverse biochemical activity. Oxygen is also much less reactive for the same reason. Also, the more electrons that an element shares with other elements, the more stable the compound becomes, or, in other words, the less reactive the element. This eliminates iron, phosphorous and sulfur from the list of the most biologically active elements in the body, leaving only sodium, potassium, magnesium and calcium. But both sodium and potassium produce very caustic and corrosive solutions and must be balanced with strong acid ions, such as chlorides, to bring their pH to the ideal 7.4. Magnesium and calcium, on the other hand, are only mildly alkaline and therefore can produce mildly alkaline solutions (pH 7.4) with a variety of ions. Thus, sodium and potassium are eliminated from the list of the most biologically active elements in the body, leaving only magnesium and calcium as contenders.

Another trait that active biological elements must have is the ability, not only to attract other nutrients, but also to readily release them as the body requires. Both magnesium and calcium have two electrons in their outer electron orbitals; magnesium has two electrons in its outer third orbital, and calcium has two electrons in its outer fourth orbital, which is farther from its positive nucleus than magnesium's outer third orbital. This makes calcium's electrons much more loosely bound. Thus, both magnesium and calcium have the same number of electrons (two negative charges each) to attract positive nutrients, but, because magnesium's electrons are more strongly bound to its nucleus, it has more difficulty liberating them, along with their attached nutrients. Thus, *calcium has the chemical flexibility needed to be the body's most biologically active mineral nutrient.*

There are numerous other reasons why calcium predominates so readily over the other elements in biological importance. Calcium, or *calx*, has been known since the time of the Romans as a strong building material, with much of the calcium being both removable and replaceable without the structure

95

collapsing. This is one of the most important properties in the human body, as it prevents the bodies of the middle aged to elderly, most of whom are calcium deficient, from collapsing. Another important property is calcium's ability to behave like an octopus and bind to several different elements at once. This makes *calcium the body's glue,* holding it together. It also allows it to bind and bunch up long proteins so that they can form the snake coil rosette that regulates the entrance to each human cell. Calcium also makes the best human battery. Of all the mineral nutrients, calcium requires the least ionization to produce voltage. For example, the 70 millivolt potential difference between the cell's interior and exterior fluids, which is required to open the nutrient channel so that the cell can be fed, can be produced with only 507 parts per million of calcium, versus 933 of potassium. This is probably why the body chooses calcium for the important task of producing the voltage that stimulates your heart muscles, causing it *to beat* and to pump blood. Thus, when it comes to the body's choice *calcium is number one.*

With all of the important biological duties of calcium that have previously been mentioned, it would be hard to believe that calcium could have an even more important duty, but it does: calcium is crucial in maintaining the pH of the body fluids at 7.4, and therefore, it is *crucial to the prevention of disease.* It does this by binding with phosphates, thereby liberating and allowing magnesium, sodium and potassium to make alkaline (high pH) salts as well as mild *chemical buffers* in the pH 7.7 range. A chemical buffer, such as sodium bicarbonate (baking soda), is a compound that allows its fluid to maintain a constant pH as long as it is not totally consumed by chemical reactions. For example, even if acid is introduced to the fluid containing sodium bicarbonate, the pH will remain a constant 7.7.

And, as if this was not enough of a contribution to maintaining a good pH, calcium not only liberates mineral nutrients for other duties, but it does it in such a way so as to produce its own chemical buffer, *calcium (mono) ortho-phosphate*, which, in combination with calcium bicarbonate, becomes a crucial component at holding the extracellular fluids in the healthy 7.4 pH range. Remember, not only does maintaining these healthy pH blue body fluids help to prevent disease, but it also provides the human cells with the capability of converting glucose into the four nucleotides for DNA replication, which is *crucial to both body repair and staying young in appearance.*

In a quote from the book, *The Role of Calcium in the Biological System* (1985, page 149, CRC Press), biochemical researchers state that *it is the calcium ion that triggers life*: "*Upon fertilization of the human egg by a sperm, two ion fluxes occur: the first is an initial surge of calcium ions, and the second, an influx of hydrogen resulting in the net alkalization (raising the pH) of the fluid within the egg which is necessary to initiate DNA synthesis and cell division.*" Thus, calcium fires the first shot in life, and one day it may be proven that it also fires the last shot.

Also in 1985, biochemical researchers Carifoli and Pennistion found that *a common trigger* precipitates biological events as diverse as the contraction of a muscle and the secretion of a hormone: *the trigger is a minute flux of calcium ions.*

By 1986, biochemical researchers Moolnaar, Defize and Delaat had found that, "A *sustained increase in cytoplasmic pH* (the fluids inside the cell become caustic) *and a rise in the calcium ion concentration of the cell fluids was a necessary function of DNA synthesis and cell division.*" Thus, calcium mineral deficiency inhibits natural growth and body repair.

By 1988, biochemist Marvin P. Thompson, in summarizing the research done to date on the biochemistry of calcium, stated that *"...calcium is the major regulatory ion in all living organisms, interest in calcium is logarithmically increasing, and calcium-related disorders are enormous."*

The Tucson Cancer Center reported recently in the *Journal of the National Cancer Institute* that "*a diet high in wheat bran or calcium may reduce the risk of colorectal cancer by soaking up bile acids believed to spur the tumors.*"

Even the food industry has begun to recognize the importance of calcium nutrition to human health. Advertisements extolling the high content of calcium, in such consumables as milk, fortified orange juice, and Tums® antacid, are commonplace today. However, the problem of recognition of importance is not enough. It is no good consuming mineral nutrients if the body just turns around and expels most of them. Vitamin and mineral supplements are a necessity to ensure, not only that the required amount of mineral nutrient is consumed, but also that the nutrients are absorbed into the body.

In 1915, the introduction of the refrigerator allowed fresh dairy products to always be readily available. By 1978, the average American teenager was consuming 50 gallons of milk each year while also, unfortunately, consuming 21 gallons of nutrition-robbing soft drinks. Tragically, by 1994, the amount of milk consumed had dropped to 33 gallons (a shocking 34% decrease) while the soft drinks had risen to 63 gallons (a staggering 300% increase). This has led to an impending health crisis. Soft drinks should be banned from your refrigerator. The author hopes that the reader, having prevailed through this technical chapter and now understanding why calcium is the **king of the bioelements**, will be inspired enough to go and get a glass of milk, or a cup of yogurt, or a glass of fortified orange juice before continuing with this book.

CHAPTER THIRTEEN

CAN CALCIUM CURE CANCER?

In 1931, Otto Warburg won the Nobel Prize in medicine for his discovery that cancer was anaerobic: cancer occurs in the absence of free oxygen as innocuous as this discovery might seem, it is actually a startling and significant finding worthy of a Nobel Prize. What it basically means is that cancer is caused by a lack of free oxygen in the body and therefore, whatever causes this to occur is the cause of all cancers.

In chemistry, alkali solutions (pH over 7.0) tend to absorb oxygen, while acids (pH under 7.0) tend to expel oxygen. For example, a mild alkali can absorb over 100 times as much oxygen as a mild acid. Therefore, when the body becomes acidic by dropping below pH 7.0 (note: all body fluids, except for stomach and urine, are supposed to be mildly alkaline at pH 7.4), oxygen is driven out of the body thereby, according to Nobel Prize winner Otto Warburg, induces cancer. Stomach fluids must remain acidic to digest food, and urine must remain acidic to remove wastes from the body. Blood is the exception. Blood must always remain at an alkaline pH 7.4 so that it can retain its oxygen. When adequate mineral consumption is in the diet, the blood is supplied the crucial minerals required to maintain an alkaline pH of 7.4. However, when insufficient mineral consumption is in the diet, the body is forced to rob Peter (other body fluids) to pay Paul (the blood). In doing so, it removes crucial minerals, such as calcium, from the saliva, spinal fluids, kidneys, liver, etc., in order to maintain the blood at pH 7.4. This causes the demineralized fluids and organs to become acidic and therefore anaerobic, thus inducing not only cancer, but a host of other degenerative diseases, such as heart disease, diabetes, arthritis, lupus, etc.

Everyone knows that the human body is made up of 78% water by weight, and that water is hydrogen and oxygen gases. When nitrogen gas and carbon in the form of carbon dioxide and methane gases are added, the total gas in the body by weight becomes over 95%. Almost half of the remaining 5% that makes up the human body and controls all biological functions is the mineral calcium.

No other mineral is capable of performing as many biological functions as is calcium. This amazing mineral provides the electrical energy for the heart to beat and for all muscle movement. It is the calcium ion that is responsible for feeding every cell. It does this by latching onto seven nutrient molecules and one water molecule and pulling them through the nutrient channel. It then detaches its load and returns to repeat the process. Another important biological job for calcium is DNA replication, which is crucial for maintaining youth and a healthy body. Calcium ions are indispensable for DNA replication ("Calcium in the Action of Growth Factors," W.H. Moolenaar, L.K. Defize, and S.W. Delaat, 1986 *Calcium and the Cell*, Wiley) which is the basis for all body repair. It can only occur *"on a substrate of calcium"* (*The Role of Calcium in Biological Systems*, Albert Lehniger, Professor of Medical Science, John Hopkins University, Volume I, CRC Press). Thus, low calcium means low body repair and premature aging. As important as all these and hundreds of other biological functions of calcium are to human health, none is more important than the job of pH control. Calcium to acid, is like water to a fire. Calcium quickly destroys oxygen-robbing acid in the body's fluids. Thus, the more calcium, the more oxygen, and therefore, the less cancer and other degenerative disease.

This information then begs the question, "How much calcium is necessary?" The answer can readily be determined by examining the diet of millions of people around the world who consume over 100 times our Recommended Daily Allowance (RDA), and who suffer the side effects of living 40 years longer than we do, of aging at half the rate that we do, and of being devoid of cancer, heart disease, mental disorders, diabetes, arthritis and all other degenerative diseases. Almost all of these people, the Armenians, Azerbaijanis and Georgians in Russia, the Tibetans, the Hunzas of Northern Pakistan, the Vilcabamba Indians in Ecuador, the Bamas in China and the Titicacas in Peru live at high altitudes above 8,000 feet. Their only source of water is melting glaciers, and the glacial water is turbid and white with ground up rock. Each quart of this water contains over 17,000 milligrams of calcium along with other minerals and 60 trace metals. These cultures drink several quarts each day and the water-fertilized crops are also loaded with calcium and other nutrients. The only long-living and disease-free culture that does not live above an altitude of 8,000 feet is the Okinawan.

Millions of Okinawans live in the southern coral islands of Japan, with the longest life expectancy in the world, while mainland Japan is just 77 years. The Okinawans live on islands made of coral reefs, which are mainly calcium. The Okinawans discovered over 500 years ago that feeding coral sand that is produced from the weathering of the reefs to the chickens and cows results in twice as many eggs and twice as much milk. They also found that when the coral sand is used as a fertilizer, crops increase by as much as threefold. When they finally – 500 years ago – began to consume the coral sand themselves, all of the underutilized doctors were forced to leave the islands. This was known in Japanese history as the Japanese Exodus.

The early European explorers discovered their secret and hauled shiploads of the calcium-rich coral sands back to Europe. In Madrid, Spain, the historic monument of the world's first drugstore contains rows of shelves labeled, *"coral calcium from Okinawa Japan."* Today, millions of people all over the world consume coral calcium, and as a result, there are millions of medical testimonials.

The phenomenon of preventing and reversing degenerative disease through the consumption of large amounts of minerals and vitamins did not go unnoticed by men of medicine. Hundreds of years ago, European doctors were prescribing coral calcium and other nutrients to their patients.

In the 1950s, Dr. Carl Reich discovered that his patients were able to "cure themselves" of almost all degenerative diseases by consuming several times the RDA of calcium, magnesium, vitamin D and other nutrients. Dr. Reich was the first North American doctor to prescribe "mega doses" of minerals and vitamins to his patients, and is considered by many to be the father of preventive medicine. By the 1980s, Dr. Reich had cured thousands, but had lost his license for explaining that the consumption of mineral nutrients, such as calcium, could prevent cancer and a host of other diseases. This concept was considered "too simple" to be accepted by the medical wisdom of the day. However, by the late 1990s, other medical men of wisdom were also discovering that calcium supplements could indeed reverse cancer. The October 13, 1998 issue of *The New York Times* published an article entitled **"Calcium Takes Its Place As a Superstar of Nutrients,"** in which it reports that a study published in the *Journal of the American Medical Association* reported that "increasing calcium induced normal development of the epithelia cells and might also prevent cancer in such organs as the breast, prostate and pancreas." It also reported that the *American Journal of Clinical Nutrition* published that "virtually no major organ system escapes calcium's influence," and that a research team from the University of Southern California found "adding calcium to the diet lowered the blood pressure in 110 black teenagers."

The January 14, 1999 issue of the *Phoenix Republic* wrote in an article entitled, **"Calcium Reduces Tumors,"** that *The New England Journal of Medicine* reported, "Adding calcium to the diet can keep you from getting tumors in your large intestine." Then the February 1999 issue of *Reader's Digest* wrote in an article entitled, **"The 'Superstar' Nutrient,"** that *The Journal of the American Medical Association* published, "When the participant's consumption reached 1,500 milligrams of calcium a day, cell growth in the colon improved toward normal (this means that the cancer was reversed)." The *Digest* also reported that the Metabolic Bone Center at St. Luke's Hospital believes that "a chronic deficiency of calcium is largely responsible for premenstrual syndrome (PMS)" and that "a lot of women are avoiding the sun and their vitamin D levels may be very low." In the same article, the *Digest* reported that "in 1997, the large, federally financed trial found that a diet containing 1,200 milligrams of calcium significantly lowered blood pressure in adults." Then the May 3, 1999 edition of *US World News Report* wrote in an article entitled, **"Calcium's Powerful Mysterious Ways"** that "Researchers are increasingly finding that the humble mineral calcium plays a major role in warding off major illnesses from high blood pressure to colon cancer," and that "You name the disease, and calcium is beginning to have a place there," (David McCarron, a nephrologists at Oregon Health Sciences University). Unfortunately, most doctors have not heard the news that their own journals and major popular newspapers and magazines are reporting that natural supplements—especially calcium—can cure and prevent disease.

It is interesting to also note that a study by the Albert Einstein College of Medicine reported in the April 2000 journal,

Nature, that "free radicals have also been linked to the destruction of cells in diabetics, triggering blindness, kidney failure and cardiovascular disease." Free radicals, which also cause Parkinson's disease, are all positively charged and are destroyed entry into a negatively charged alkaline body, the result of sunshine and calcium.

The scientific evidence that calcium is the key to good and long health is overwhelming. Just 20 years ago, any doctor making the claim that calcium supplements could cure cancer would lose his license. Dr. Carl Reich lost his license for making this claim which the medical authorities of the day branded as *"too simplistic."* Yet today, the doctor's own Journals – *The New England Journal of Medicine, The Journal of the American Medical Association*, and the *American Journal of Clinical Nutrition* – are all making the claim that calcium supplements can reverse cancer and that virtually no organ escapes calcium's influence. These journals have been quoted in our popular and respectable newspapers and magazines. We have come a long way, and still have a long way to go. At present, it is almost impossible to find a doctor who is aware of these scientific findings. Therefore, we must get the doctors to read their own journals and then do an almost impossible task: get the AMA and the FDA to do their jobs and endorse these scientific findings. When this finally occurs, over 90% of disease will be irradiated, thereby eliminating massive pain and suffering, and we will be well on our way to *curing America.*

So then, what are the nutrients that the body needs to cure itself? The answer begins with calcium. There is no such thing as a bad calcium nutrient. All calcium nutrients are good for producing a healthy body; however, some are better than others. For example, the consumption of coral calcium provides adequate calcium, magnesium and dozens of trace minerals for absorption by the body. Some calcium nutrients, such as calcium carbonate, are difficult for the body to absorb. This does not mean that they are not good, but rather that there are better choices. Also, there is no such thing as bad coral calcium from Okinawa; they are all *miracle minerals*. However, some are better than others. The Japanese grade the coral based on magnesium content. The more magnesium a coral has, the higher it is graded. Consuming coral calcium can be classified in the same category as breathing as both fill the body with life-sustaining oxygen. Most suppliers of coral calcium instruct you to take two to three capsules each day. But this is for *maintaining* good health. When you are sick, it is best to double-up to four to six per day. If you are really sick, with a disease such as cancer, lupus, diabetes, etc., it is best to triple-up to six to nine per day. The author has been told by many that a few months on the larger dose coral has successfully terminated their cancer, lupus, multiple sclerosis and numerous other incurable diseases. Of course, all of these people exposed themselves to sunshine, and to a host of other nutrients as well as the coral calcium.

Of course, other nutrients are also required – the most important being exposure to sunshine. Sun on the skin produces inisotol triphospate to regulate mineral disposition in the body, and it also produces vitamin D, which allows the intestine to absorb large amounts of nutrients. The ultraviolet radiation from the sun striking the eyes stimulates the pituitary, pineal and hypothymus glands at the back of the eye to regulate the production of many hormones such as melatonin, seritonin and calcium-regulating calcitonin. Thus, lack of sunshine on the body is responsible for a host of diseases, especially cancer. This sounds like a controversial statement, but not when you look at the facts. The cancer-free, Black African is naked in the sun all day while the Black American – who avoids the sun like the plague – has three times the cancer rate of the sun-worshipping White American. There is twice as much breast cancer in the northern states as in the sunny southern states. Prostate cancer goes up almost 300% from the sunny Mexican border to the northern Canadian border. When exposure to the sun does trigger skin cancer, the victim is usually a white albino who already has five other mineral-deficiency-induced diseases, and is well on the way to developing the sixth.

Other important nutrient sources are multivitamins, which can be purchased inexpensively in all major stores. The instructions on the bottle may say to take one each day; however, the many cultures around the world that never get sick take about 100 times the amounts that is recommended in America. This means that you should take several every day – the author recommends at least six per day – as by the millions, these people have proven that there is no such thing as too much when it comes to vitamins and minerals. There is however, one exception, and that is large amounts of *liquid calcium* that can lead to hypercalcemia if the body is not exposed to sunlight for at least one hour each day. Large quantities of coral calcium do not require sunshine, as no amount of coral calcium can cause hypercalcemia. Also, trace minerals can be found in most health stores. Once again, the instructions will say one per day, but six per day is recommended. Vitamin D is also necessary to ensure the absorption of nutrients. A minimum of 5,000 IUs is suggested. Extra boron, selenium, chromium, zinc, vitamin A, vitamin E and cesium is also recommended.

Although almost all degenerative diseases can be prevented and cured nutritionally if given enough time, people are always asking, *"What can I do if I am terminal?"* A terminal cancer patient, for example, may be cured over a six-month period by consuming the proper nutrients, but may only have three weeks to live. This situation requires a more potent nutrient treatment, such as cesium chloride, for example. Cesium chloride is a natural salt, and where it is found, cancer does not exist. This is because cesium is the most caustic mineral that exists, and when it enters the body, it seeks out all of the acidic cancer hotspots, dousing the fire of cancer, thereby terminating the cancer within days. Also, when dimethyl sulfoxide (DMSO) is rubbed near a painful cancer, the pain is removed and the DMSO causes the cesium to penetrate the cancer tumor much faster, thereby terminating the cancer much faster. DMSO is an approved drug in 125 countries around the world, and 600 million people have used it therapeutically. Larger doses of vitamin D will cause the body to alkalize faster, bringing a speedy end to the cancer. Otto Warburg's oxygen respiration enzyme formula (Oxy-Plus) has also been proven to be effective against cancer. Dr. Karl Folker discovered CoQ10 in the 1960s while working for the giant pharmaceutical company, Merck. He found it to eliminate cancerous tumors in the breast, lungs and stomach *(Biochemical and Biophysical Research Communications*, March 30, 1994.) And finally, gold metal absorbed by the body has been found effective in recovering from cancer.

The following program has worked for some with cancer:

1. Consume 6 coral calcium capsules each day: 2 in morning, 2 in afternoon and 2 at night.
2. Consume 100 grams of cesium chloride at 3 grams each day: one gram morning, noon and night, total 33 days.
3. Consume 100 milligrams of CoQ10 each day for 30 days.
4. Consume one Oxy-Plus (500 mg) three times each day.
5. Apply DMSO gel to skin nearest the cancer (or nearest to pain) twice a day.
6. Apply gold gel to skin nearest the cancer once each day.
7. Consume 6 vitamin D tablets (5,000 IUs) each day: 2 in the morning, 2 in the afternoon and 2 at night.
8. Eat two bananas, and/or two large potatoes, two glasses of milk or two glasses of orange juice and eat raisons, tomatoes, spinach or broccoli every day (all contain lots of potassium, magnesium and calcium).
9. Expose your skin and face to at least two hours of sunshine every day with no skin block and no glasses (allows for the production of inositol triphosphate, calcitonin and vitamin D to help regulate crucial minerals such as calcium). Sun exposure is mandatory, even with skin cancer.

Note:

1. This program will help to alkalize the body's fluids, resulting in the toxins, which are adhered to the cell surface, detaching themselves and entering the blood. The body will recognize the toxins as foreign invaders and respond by attacking them, possibly causing flu-like symptoms such as headaches, stomachaches and diarrhea. This is called "detoxing," and it means that the body is ridding itself of cancer-inducing compounds.

2. After the cesium has been consumed (33 days), the cancer can be benign (only a biopsy can prove this). Continue taking all of the other nutrients except for the DMSO, which should only be used for pain control.

The author has witnessed numerous people with terminal cancers who have employed the above program successfully. In the author's web site (**www.barefootscureamerica.com**), and in the Testimonials section of this book, numerous testimonials are provided by prestigious Americans.

Alkalizing the body with nutrition allows the body to cure itself, even from previously incurable diseases. Nobel Prize winner, Otto Warburg complained in 1966 that because the agnostics were in control, millions of men and women would have to die needlessly from cancer. Today the agnostics are still in control, but their control has weakened substantially, due to information exchange by computers and the Internet. One does not have to be a rocket scientist to read simple articles in reputable newspapers and magazines, quoting the doctors' own journals that are all saying that disease can be cured by diet. The time is ripe to end the needless suffering, pain and death caused by curable degeneration diseases such as cancer and heart disease. The time has come to *cure America.*

CHAPTER FOURTEEN

THE EARTH NUTRIENT

By now the reader must feel that he or she is swimming in an ocean of technical facts. The good news is that you are very buoyant in salt water, so the ocean is the easiest place to swim. In other words, if you have made it this far, you have been capable of understanding *the cause of disease* – something that hitherto was supposed to be well beyond your grasp. The other good news is that the worst is over. From here on it gets much easier. Once you understand the cause, prevention and cure, and the recipes for good health, become more obvious. However, before the recipes are described, it is necessary to look at one more of the ingredients, the nutrient, Earth.

When the father of medicine, Hippocrates, said, "*Sunshine and fresh air must be considered as good food,*" he was referring to the medicinal properties of both. Although modern medicine wholeheartedly agrees about the medicinal properties of fresh air, it is astounding that modern medicine seems to disagree with Hippocrates on the medicinal properties of sunshine, as all who will listen are warned to wear skin creams to block the sunshine which *causes skin cancer.* Of course, as has been demonstrated, *sunshine is not the cause of skin cance*r, and the verdict is still out regarding the potential long-term damage to human health that may be caused by the use of *sun blockers*.

The word "*fresh*" when applied to air means negatively charged. Thus, when the air feels fresh after a rain, technically, the air is negatively charged. In fact, after a rain, the air contains thousands of times more electrons than it did before the rain. This is caused by water rubbing the air, resulting in the water becoming positively charged and the air negatively charged. If this is so, and it is, why do humans feel so good after a rain?

The answer lies in the fact that the human body is a beehive of bioelectrical activity. The body fluids are alkaline and therefore negatively charged. As the charge is consumed – initiating biochemical reactions – the body reacts to try to produce more electrons. Thus, when the fresh air bathes the human body with electrons, the strain on the body to produce more electrons is relieved and biochemical activity is stimulated, resulting in a good feeling. On the other hand, ill winds, which are dry, positively charged air, suppress biochemical activity. And so, fresh air is indeed a nutrient and *Hippocrates was right!*

Regarding modern medicine's misconception of sunshine, the only answer would be numerous sabbaticals spent reading biochemical texts in the library. But for now, a quick recap: First, the sun produces photosynthetic (light-induced) chemicals in the skin, the most important being *vitamin D*. Another, almost equally important biochemical product of photosynthesis is *inisotol triphospate (INSP-3)*, an active vitamin-calcium-releasing agent.

One question that should be asked is, "Why are blood veins found near the surface of the skin?" The answer is, "sunshine," as *hemoglobin* (the component of the blood which carries oxygen) *is excitonic*, just like the chlorophyll in plants.

110

When these molecules are stimulated by specific frequencies in the light spectrum, electron pairs (like the famous **Cooper Pair** of electrons responsible for superconductivity) are formed along with their created "positive hole." The combination of the electron pairs or electron couplet and the associated positive hole is known as an **exciton**. This incredibly long-lasting combination of electron pair, in a high and congested energy level and positive hole, can then travel the surface of the molecule. Occasional collisions (exciton fusion) with other excitons then liberates energy in the form of electrons (which is sub-atomic power without any radiation). Both chlorophyll and hemoglobin have similar chemical structure with one basic difference: chlorophyll has magnesium in the center and hemoglobin has iron. The exciton-produced electrons provide energy for the plants to create carbohydrates from carbon dioxide and water (a process known as *the secret of life*), and in the blood, these electrons satisfy the cravings of the electron-hungry biochemical reactions. Unfortunately, nuclear radiation, which can penetrate more deeply than sunlight into the body, is also capable of producing electrons from the positively charged excitonic carcinogen molecules, which were attached to the negatively charged cell surface. With their positive charge now neutralized, these carcinogens become detached, freeing them to participate in the mutation of the cells (cancer). **Wow!** The chapter begins with a promise of diminishing technical concepts, and now the reader has been introduced to a new form of *subatomic power*!

Another question that should be asked is, *"Why are both the hypothalamus* (part of the brain that regulates energy balance through control of appetite, sleep, body temperature, regulation of sexual function and control of water balance) *and the pituitary gland* (known as the master gland, as it produces a host of hormones) *situated directly behind the eyes?"* The answer, of course, is because they both react to light stimulation. There is a whole new science called *photobiology* that is based on

111

light stimulation of the body. For example, being in a yellow room stimulates people to learn, and being in a pink room can quickly calm those who are excited. Sunlight stimulation causes the pituitary gland to direct the parathyroid glands to produce *the hormone, calcitonin*, which results in the body removing its required calcium from the cells. Lack of sunshine stimulation results in the production of the *parathyroid hormone*, which results in the body removing its required calcium from the bones, thereby weakening them. The list of biochemical stimulation by sunshine is very extensive. Thus, sunshine is a nutrient and once again, *Hippocrates, the father of medicine, was right*!

It seems that the non-edible nutrients provided by the Earth—except for sunshine—are all invisible. No discussion about the importance of the biochemistry of the Earth's nutrients would be complete without a discussion about the total environment in which the body's many biochemical reactions takes place. For example, it is well known that pressure and temperature – two invisible physical parameters – can affect the outcome of many chemical reactions. Two such examples are the application of heat to acids dramatically speeding up digestion, and the application of a vacuum to a liquid speeding up the chemical production of gases. Both pressure and temperature effects have been documented for hundreds of years. What has not been documented or clearly understood is the effect that electromagnetic fields have on biochemical reactions. The laws of physics state that with every magnetic field, there is an associated electrical field. Electrical fields definitely affect biochemical reactions which are all based on electron transfers. The Earth's magnetic field is therefore an example of an invisible nutrient. It is a nutrient because it is an essential ingredient in stimulating or retarding biochemical activity. Of course, the concept of magnetics affecting human health will once again bring out cries of *"quackery* and *snake oil salesman!"* But of course, with a world of evidence and experts supporting the concepts, it is absolutely amazing that it could have been suppressed so long from the American public.

To begin with, let us use some very basic and simple logic. As Dr. Becker would say, *"the body is electric!"* A myriad of bioelectrical reactions occur every second. Dr. Becker discovered that a stream of electrons would flow from the new wounds of both animals and plants. He found that this electrical *current of injury* could be correlated to both the extent of the injury and to reparative growth. Dr. Becker also found that the rate of regeneration of limbs on animals that could regenerate severed limbs was proportional to the current of injury. Thus, armed with these new scientific facts, he began to experiment by artificially superimposing electrical currents on the wounds of animals, such as dogs, which do not have regeneration capability. Dr. Becker successfully regrew limbs on several species of animals, but was denied permission to experiment on humans. Instead, the medical establishment had his research funds revoked. There can be no doubt that in the next century, Dr. Becker's research will lead to the *regeneration of human limbs.*

Bioelectrical reactions in the human body can easily be measured with electronic instrumentation. Their associated magnetic fields are more difficult to measure. The laws of physics tell us that if these magnetic fields are superimposed by another magnetic field, then the result will be a changed bioelectrical field, resulting in altered voltages and thereby altered biochemical reactions. Thus, because each biochemical reaction depend on specific voltages at specific times – which are being altered by a superimposing magnetic field – the *superimposing* (invisible) *magnetic field does change the body's chemistry.*

In early space flights, up to 8% of the astronauts' bones decalcified (*space osteoporosis*) after only a few weeks in orbit. The spacecraft's rapid motion, cutting across the Earth's magnetic lines of force, caused electrical currents to be induced in the astronauts' bodies (law of physics: when a conductor cuts across magnetic lines of force, an electric current is induced in the conductor). Although the human body is a poor conductor, only small electrical currents are necessary to produce osteoporosis. This is because the process of human cell division, which involves the duplication of all of the cell's DNA and chromosomes which are then distributed equally to all of the cells, takes *exactly 24 hours!* This implies that tissue repair is in cyclic harmony with Earth's rotation, and the astronauts, rotating Earth approximately every hour, were out of harmony with their cell replication. The problem was solved by the Russians, who used pulsed magnetic fields at the Schumann rate of resonance which induced – from outside of the body – normal biochemical electrical currents inside of the body.

Another fact of physics is that the north pole of a magnet is negative, and the south pole is positive. The explanation for the negative fresh air stimulating biochemical reactions in the body applies in this case. Thus, the north pole of a magnet is preferable for stimulating good health. After decades of stalling and refusing to budge, the American medical authorities finally relented, and – yielding to public pressure – gave their rare approval in 1979 for American hospitals to use pulsed magnetic fields to stimulate bone growth. Currently, every major hospital in America employs pulsed magnetic fields to stimulate bone healing, which reduces the time required to heal the bones to about *one tenth the time normally* required. The use of magnetic therapy for other ailments – while used extensively by other cultures – is still frowned on in America. Most Americans would be astounded to learn that currently, one out of every twenty Japanese sleep on magnetic beds. The same is happening in Germany. This includes thousands of highly trained medical doctors who *claim* that not only do their ailments appear to be *curing themselves* while they sleep, but also, they arise from their sleep with *unusual energy*.

114

One interesting fact that is emerging from the human magnetic bed experiment, is that *the body fluids become alkaline after only a few hours of exposure* and then return to their pre-exposure acidic state a few hours later. For example, those with an acidic saliva pH of 6.0 prior to sleeping on a magnetic bed, awake with an alkaline pH of 7.4 after a good night's sleep on a magnetic bed (north poles towards the body). This induced, high-pH-body-fluid state while exposed to a magnetic field, means that the body is not only *healing itself*, but that the body is also *absorbing more oxygen*. Raising the pH of the external cell fluids also raises the potential difference (voltage) between the internal and external cell fluids, thereby allowing the cell's nutrient channels to function more efficiently. The internal cell fluids thus become more alkaline, which *stimulates the production of the four DNA nucleotides* from the glucose nutrient, thereby ensuring replication of the cell's DNA. This explains the feeling of exhilaration and energy experienced after sleeping on a magnetic bed.

Now, the question arises, *How does a magnetic field raise the pH of the body's fluids?* It has been known since the turn of the century that passing liquid through a high-gauss (one gauss is one magnetic line per square centimeter) magnetic field causes the pH of the liquid to rise. Ships are equipped with these devices, which prevent scale buildup in their boilers. As scale is calcium carbonate, passing water containing calcium bicarbonate through a magnetic field must convert the bicarbonate to hydroxides, thereby (because no carbonate anions are present in the liquid) preventing the production of the precipitous calcium carbonate, known as boiler slag. The magnetic field, with its associated electrical field, reorganizes the calcium bicarbonate so that all of the positive atoms are pulled to the negative north pole and the negative atoms are pulled towards the positive south pole. Thus, the *bicarbonate is forced to bend, and the stress causes it to break* forming one calcium hydroxide molecule and two carbon dioxide gas molecules. Calcium hydroxide cannot form scale, and in the blood and body fluids, it causes the pH to become alkaline, and therefore, healthy.

Unfortunately, not all magnetic fields are healthy. Those generated by the Earth are necessary to maintain good health. However, many magnetic fields generated by man can be very harmful to human health. Electrobiologists have determined that, since humans are cyclic creatures (cell division cycle time occurs every 24 hours, or every one rotation of the Earth), frequencies most detrimental to biological functions occur in the *extremely low frequency (ELF)* range between 1 to 100 cycles per second. Unfortunately, most electrical power supplies are at 60 cycles per second, which is in the middle of this range. The *current of injury* resulting in the healing of wounds is only 0.00006 volts or 60 microvolts.

Exposure to radio waves at 16 hertz (or cycles per second) dramatically increases the flow of calcium from the brain cells, interfering with the impulse transmission, changing brain function and causing confusion. Russian scientists found that dogs could be made to run in circles chasing their tails, much like they expected the American generals to do in war time when they would be exposed to this technology they did not understand. The offspring of rats exposed to one month of 60-cycles-per-second electric fields, simulating ground level under typical electrical power transmission lines, showed both *stunted growth and high mortality rates*, especially among males. ELF fields have also been shown to change brainstem levels of the neurotransmitter acetylcholine. Human cancer cells exposed to 60-cycles-per-second electromagnetic fields for no more than 24 hours experienced a sixfold increase in their growth rate in just one week. And the list goes on. Thus, ELF fields, the major source of *electropollution*, superimposed over our natural bioelectric field, can have serious negative health consequences. Ionic calcium, the main generator of the body's bioelectric fields can be adversely affected by the

116

ELF fields emanating from common household appliances. This could lead to over 147 different diseases. Despite this evidence, as was the case with the Dr. Semmelweis's invisible germs, the authorities cannot come to grips with something that they cannot see and something that they were not responsible for discovering, and therefore, they are in a *constant state of denial*.

In summary, the Earth can provide both *visible and invisible non-edible nutrients* necessary for good health. Earth's magnetic fields, which help regulate our biochemical functions, have gone from *4-gauss* (magnetic lines per square centimeter) at the time of Christ, to currently less than *1-gauss*. Our ignorance of these mechanisms has resulted in an Earth that emanates many invisible electrical pollutants that are very harmful to human and animal health. When, within the next 1,000 years, Earth's magnetic field becomes *0-gauss*, what will be the consequences to human biochemistry if we continue to keep our heads in the sand, ignoring these basic facts of life.

Note: Earth's magnetic field is generated by the electrical currents produced electrostatically by Earth's mantle moving at a different speed than Earth's molten core. When the mantle moves faster than the molten core, the flow of the electrical current in a westerly direction—causes the magnetic pole to be in the north (left-hand rule used by electrical buffs for establishing polarity). Likewise, when the mantle moves slower than the molten core, the flow of electrical current will be in an easterly direction, causing the magnetic pole to be in the south. Every million or so years the magnetic poles *"flip."* When the mantle and core are moving at the same speed, no static electricity is produced, and therefore no magnetic pole exists. The changing speed of Earth's mantle relative to Earth's molten core is caused by the cyclic changes in the orbit of the solar system. The torque on Earth, generated by the solar system's elliptical orbit through space and by the positioning of other celestial objects, dictates the changing speed of the mantle, and thereby the intensity of the electro-static currents and the associated magnetic field. When the solar system reaches the two shallowest points of its orbit, no torque is exerted, and therefore no electrical current and no magnetic field exist. At one of the points, the mantle starts to go faster than the core; at the other point the mantle starts to go slower than the core. This causes the *flipping* of the magnetic poles. When the solar system reaches the two outer extended limits of its elliptical path, the most torque is generated and the greatest electrical current with the largest magnetic field is generated. As long as the solar system is in its elliptical orbit, the cycles will continue.

The question arises, "*Will we soon have to produce artificial magnetic fields for the human race to survive as a species?*" Our ignorance of these basic biological mechanisms has resulted in our not using Earth's gifts in a positive manner while we produce many invisible electrical pollutants that are very harmful to human and animal health.

CHAPTER FIFTEEN

THE MAGIC MUSHROOM

What is a *"magic mushroom"*? Although millions of people around the world use magic mushrooms, there are only a few people in America who even know what a magic mushroom is. To begin with, the name is a double misnomer, it is not magic and it is not a mushroom. What is being referred to is a bacterial fungi yeast "paddy" that looks like a floating, dirty, uncooked pancake as it hovers over, and is nurtured by, a solution of sugared tea water. Within days it will have grown into two, back-to-back paddies, stuck together, and the sugared tea water will have been converted into one of the most nutritious and refreshing drinks ever created. In other words, this magic mushroom produces a lightly fermented tea, which is known worldwide as *kombucha*. Although the magic mushroom has explainable scientific merit, it has two qualities that make it unacceptable to Western medicine: *it is very inexpensive to make, and it is **very effective in the fight against disease**.*

Where then, did this magic mushroom come from? Kombucha is an ancient homemade folk remedy that is supposed to have originated in China over two thousand years ago. Then, in 415 A.D, *Emperor **Kombu*** of Japan became gravely ill. Emissaries were sent around the world seeking cures. They returned to Japan with a mushroom that produced a medicinal tea, or *"cha"* in Japanese. The Emperor recovered and lived a healthy and productive life. News of the tea, now known as *"kombucha,"* spread around the world. The magic mushroom began to bloom westward, where today, in countries such as Russia and Germany, it is a very common and popular drink for millions of people.

Of course, there are just about as many claims of the health benefits of kombucha as there are people who drink it. Such claims have brought the wrath of the medical establishments for hundreds of years, but people just keep on drinking it, and making more claims. There are just so many people claiming health benefits that it would be absolutely ludicrous to suggest that they all could be wrong. In fact, there are bundles of medical studies, relegated to the wastebaskets of the ruling medical establishments of the time that verify many, but not all, of the miraculous claims. They have their *experts* too, and that is all that is required to get an exact opposite opinion. Experts tend to be men with all of the answers *but none of the solutions*. The author's grandmother used to joke that *"Experts were all very important men who lost their 'r,'"* which would make them very *"impotent"* men. German Professor, Ulrich Beck stated that *"Whenever a motley bunch of experts, let's say five scientists, is asked some question, you will get fifteen answers, all hedged with 'yes-but, on one hand, on the other hand,' if those asked the question are any good; if they are not, you will get two or three apparently definite answers."* Professor Beck's opinion is supported by the old saying of many cultures around the world, *"the less they know, the more certain they are."* Thus, *the battle of logic* can never be won by challenging the men who have none.

The general public, on the other hand, is more conducive to logical arguments. Once the components of kombucha and its biological activities are explained, the public will both

120

understand how kombucha works to enhance health and believe many of the claims.

Kombucha could be said to be nothing more than a fermented sugar tea, and also nothing less. Teas are known worldwide to contain vitamins and nutrients, so there can be no objection about this component. Sugar on the other hand, especially the white sugar that the recipe calls for, will bring condemnation from nutritional *experts* worldwide, despite the fact that the major nutrient feeding the human cell is *the sugar, glucose*. However, their criticism will be invalid, as the white sugar used is almost totally converted by fermentation to other nutrients. *Fermentation* is the chemical change in a solution brought about by microscopic yeasts, bacteria and molds. Good things such as penicillin, cheese and wine are products of fermentation.

The good things produced by kombucha fermentation are vitamin C, the B vitamins, a small amount of alcohol (about 0.5 %), gluconic acid, glucuronic acid, lactic acid, acetic acid, oxalic acid and a few other organic acids, such as acetic acid, which ancient healers knew thousands of years ago to be *the wonder elixir for a healthier life*. Even Japan's feared Samurai warriors of years ago relied on vinegar for strength and power. Today, some believe that because of the high organic acid content, kombucha could make the body acidic, but just the opposite is true. These weak acids help dissolve nutrients and then combine with them to produce alkaline salts which raise the pH of the body's fluids. This allows the body to absorb more oxygen and ward off disease, as well as providing an environment conducive to normal biological activity. Many people who have difficulty raising the pH of their body fluids report rapid increases in the alkalinity of their pH just weeks after drinking kombucha daily. And, if that were not enough, these organic alkaline salts result in the dissolution of toxins, which then combine with glucuronic acid so that they can be expelled from the body by the kidneys. This function is usually carried out by the liver, which is often hard-pressed to both dissolve toxins and produce enough glucuronic acid to ensure their expulsion from the body. Thus, kombucha alleviates stress on the liver, which probably accounts for the thousands of documented claims about liver-ailment cures. An interesting aside: many Russians claim to never get hangovers, no matter how much vodka they drink, as long as they maintain their daily dose of Kombucha (Note: hangovers are caused by toxins in the brain).

Where do I get some kombucha? Well, first you need a magic mushroom, which can be purchased from a health food store or, because of its ability to split into two mushrooms every week, you can get one from a friend, as most people do. To make three quarts of kombucha, all you need − other than the magic mushroom − is a cup of white sugar and five tea bags. Simply put three quarts of water in a ceramic or Teflon-lined container (Note: the mushroom is sensitive to damage by contact with metal, thus do not use metal containers or spoons) and bring to a boil. Then add one cup of sugar and continue to boil for five minutes. Add five tea bags, regular store-bought tea is preferable, and let steep for ten minutes before removing them. Allow to come to room temperature. Pour your cool sugar tea into a glass container and, as fermentation requires some acid, add a half-cup of kombucha that contains suspended yeast from the previous batch, or, if you don't have any, add a couple of tablespoons full of vinegar. Now comes the most interesting, and the most crucial part. Remember that the magic mushroom is a bacterial fungi, and *it should not be touched by unclean hands*, for to do so may result in the production of foreign bacteria (foreign bacteria in any food can result in food poisoning) in your kombucha. Gently place the magic mushroom on the top of the acidified sugar tea, where it will float and immediately begin to grow. Cover the top with cheesecloth so that the fermentation can get the required oxygen, while preventing vinegar flies from nesting in the mushroom. Place in a clean, warm environment, as cooling slows down the fermentation, and uncleanliness could introduce foreign bacteria, the only real source of complaints that could make you sick. This last statement should not cause concern, because the same could be said for bacterial invasion of all foods.

Six days later, your kombucha is ready to drink, that is, if you prefer it just a little sweet. One more day of fermentation (seven days total is the usual), and it produces a drink that tastes somewhat like apple cider. If you allow a few more days of fermentation, it will become quite sour with the production of acetic acid. If you wait more than two weeks, you will have vinegar, which is both excellent and very nutritious on salads. The floating yeast is usually allowed to settle before drinking, and most people prefer to drink it cold with ice. The final result is a *delicious and inexpensive drink* (about a penny a glass) that is loaded with the nutrients the body craves.

Other questions that are frequently asked are the following:

1. How long will the mushroom last? Technically, it will grow indefinitely. However, it is recommended that, as you get a new split of mushroom each week, you dispose of the original at least every three months.

2. Can I eat the mushroom? Yes you can , and many people do, although most do not find it to be tasty.

3. How can I save several mushrooms? You can put several in sugar tea in one container and put it in your fridge, as the cool temperature will slow down the fermentation. You can also freeze the mushroom, but this must be done as quickly as possible (i.e.: put it directly on ice) so as to prevent ice crystallization from damaging the mushroom.

4. How much kombucha is it safe to drink? Many Russians drink a gallon a day, but, as kombucha helps the body to absorb nutrients, a glass at each meal is recommended.

5. How many calories does kombucha contain? Most of the

calories are in the sugar, of which there is very little left after fermentation. A teaspoon of sugar contains about 20 calories, and it is doubtful that there would be a teaspoon of sugar left in the three quarts of kombucha after seven days of fermentation.

6. Has anybody ever gotten sick from drinking kombucha? Unfortunately, the answer is "*Yes, people have gotten sick from drinking kombucha, but it was not the kombucha that made them sick.*" Foreign bacteria, which got into the mushroom because it was not – as instructed – kept in a clean environment, caused the ailments. When people get sick from eating chicken with salmonella bacteria, the salmonella is blamed as the cause, and the chicken gets a clean bill of health, as should kombucha.

7. Can I vary the recipe? Until you have established yourself as a competent kombucha gourmet, the answer is that you should not attempt to do this. There are, however, some old timers who have experimented successfully with various fruits and ports.

8. Do I have to worry about the alcohol in Kombucha? No! After seven days, the brew contains only about one half of one percent alcohol, which is the equivalent of non-alcohol wine or non-alcohol beer.

For those who seek more information on kombucha, the author recommends the following book: *Kombucha, Healthy Beverage and Natural Remedy from the Far East,* by Gunther W. Frank.

Kombucha is probably one of the most nutritious and inexpensive drinks ever discovered; it helps to both prevent and cure disease, and is, therefore, *excellent for your health*.

The author's favorite drink is kombucha that has been fortified with *coral calcium*, another nutritious health product with hundreds of years of history and health claims. Coral calcium will be discussed in detail in the next chapter.

CHAPTER SIXTEEN

RECIPES FOR HEALTH

If the reader has made it this far, he or she has become somewhat familiar with the body's fluids, the human cell, the body's requirement for nutrients, and the body's harmony with the Earth. The reader will by now understand that the cause of degenerative disease is mineral deficiency of the body, and the reader will therefore have a basic idea of how to both prevent and cure disease. But unfortunately, knowing the basics is not enough, because most people want to be told – in simple terms – exactly what to do. Thus, what they want is science to give them a recipe for good health.

The first part of these recipes include putting to use what you have learned in this book so that your body has all the mineral nutrients it requires to maintain healthy, pH 7.4, body fluids. For example, the list would be as follows:

1. Hippocrates has been proven right: *sunshine is good for your health.* Don't be afraid of the sun. The sun should be one of your best friends. Although *too much* of anything is bad for your health, the same can be said for *too little.* Sunshine will cause the photosynthesis of both vitamin D and INSP-3 in your skin, both critical to human health, as they help raise the pH of the body's fluids, thereby helping to both prevent and cure disease. It will also induce excitonic reactions in your body fluids that will supply some of the energy required to maintain good health. Before the advent of artificial light, the human body, clothed in loincloth, was exposed to many hours of direct sunshine each day. This may have been too much. Less than one hour every day may be too little.

2. Not only is sunshine good for you, but also, *sunlight is good for your health*. Unfortunately, artificial light has made a major change, for the worse, in human lifestyles. It is now possible to live without sunlight. The problem that this causes is that the body is removed from some of the Earth's nutrients. Your hypothalamus and pituitary glands require unfiltered sunlight in order to regulate your appetite, sleep, body temperature, sexual functions, water balance, and hormones –many of which regulate body nutrients. All living things need to be exposed daily to sunlight. If a plant cannot grow healthy in its environment, then, in the same environment, neither will you. The human body should have at least one hour of unfiltered (preferably no windows or eyeglasses) sunlight every day. Hippocrates would definitely agree with this, as he stated that *sunshine was good food and therefore good medicine.*

3. Once again, Hippocrates' recommendation is correct: *fresh air is good for you*. This means you must get outside. Try taking a walk after every rain shower, or in the countryside if possible, while you are exposing yourself to your friend, the sun. As many pollutants, such as carbon monoxide, are heavy, the air is usually fresher at the top of a building than on the ground.

4. Try to get outside close to the Earth, as *Earth's magnetic field is good for your health.* Your body's natural bioelectrical system evolved under the influence of the overlapping magnetic field of the Earth. Although the Earth's magnetic field is very weak, so too are many of the body's bioelectric reactions – an example being the electrical requirement for the healing of wounds is only 0.00006 volts. Today, there are too many people who remain high in buildings most of every day, insulated from the Earth's magnetic fields, Mother Nature's medicine.

5. Of course, once again Hippocrates has been proven right when he advised good food is good medicine: *eat lots of fruits and vegetables*. Both are full of vitamin and mineral nutrients, and both result in the production of alkaline salts that raise the pH of you body fluids, thereby helping to both prevent and cure disease. This may result in diarrhea some of the time, as some fruits and vegetables contain lots of the mineral nutrient, magnesium. However, remember, just as a fever is the body's way of killing virus and bacteria, diarrhea is the body's way of expelling toxins. Thus, in moderation, both may be very good for your health.

6. Don't eat more than 20 ounces of red meat each week, and avoid carbonated pop that contains high phosphates. Most foods contain an abundance of phosphates, some dramatically more than others, and phosphates tend to precipitate out mineral nutrients, causing them to pass out of the body, thereby resulting in *mineral deficiency, which causes disease*. Several major industries will be angry about this recommendation, but the facts are clear: *diet can cause disease and diet can cause death.*

7. Eat white meat and fish. White meat is both nutritious and low in the phosphates which cause mineral loss in the body. Fish is both nutritious and is also a rare source of edible vitamin D.

8. Eat nutritious, natural foods such as butter and eggs. Do not avoid these foods because of their cholesterol content, as to do so you would also to be avoiding nutrients, such as choline, which are vital to human health. Besides, cholesterol is not the *cause* of heart disease, although, like all other foods, it should be consumed in moderation.

9. Drink lots of milk and dairy products, as they contain lots of mineral nutrients and some are even fortified with vitamins.

127

The most important critical nutrient is calcium, king of the bioelements. Everyone should drink milk, and when some do not, it is because their bodies are telling them not to drink the milk due to their state of acidosis. Although the bodies of such people are desperate for calcium, their bodies prefer to get calcium from a food that does not contain more of the acid, lactic acid, that is causing their acidosis. Thus, they do not like milk. It's interesting to note that once the pH of the body fluids of these people is brought back to its normal alkaline level, they will start to crave milk. The body does know best.

10. *Drink the drink of princes and paupers, drink kombucha.* Royalty drinks kombacha because it works to prevent disease and to maintain health. The poor commoner drinks kombacha because it maintains health, it only costs a penny, and it tastes so good. The nutritious organic nutrients are a powerful method of raising the alkalinity of the body's fluids, while dissolving toxins to which the kombucha's glucuronic acid can then attach itself and expel from the body. This, in effect, is a great help to your liver and kidneys.

11. *Sleep on a magnetic bed or sit on a magnetic pad,* with the north, negative pole facing your body. This will cause the pH of your body fluids to become alkaline and cure your ailments.

12. *Get to know the nutrient content of foods that you eat.* Almost all foods currently list their nutrient contents on their packages. Table 7: Mineral Nutrient Content of Some Popular Foods should help get you started.

13. *Monitor your saliva pH and take vitamin and mineral supplements* according to Table 8: Recommended Daily Supplement Program. The saliva pH of children can respond positively to the program within days, the middle aged may take weeks to a few months, and the elderly may take up to a year or more to become a healthy caustic blue.

Table 7: Mineral Nutrient Content of Some Popular Foods

Food (type)	Serving (amount)	calcium	magnesium	potassium
Yogurt, low fat	8 oz. cup	314	25	300
Ice cream	4 oz. serving	100	12	150
Orange juice, fortified	8 oz. glass	300	---	467
Milk, skim	8 oz. glass	302	33	382
Cheese	1 oz.. slice	174	15	198
Salmon, canned	3 oz. serving	167	25	272
Tomato	6 oz. (one)	5	19	491
Asparagus	2 oz. serving	10	---	110
Celery	2 oz. stick	21	6	158
Lettuce	2 oz. leaf	12	6	159
Cabbage	4 oz. serving	51	19	273
Green beans	2 oz. serving	25	---	110
Corn	4 oz. serving	4	---	314
Peas	4 oz. serving	29	12	150
Broccoli	4 oz. serving	108	---	478
Spinach	4 oz. serving	111	67	557
Green barley essence	3 gm, teaspoon	33	68	264
Onion	2 oz. slice	23	5	78
Potato	8 oz. serving	30	---	334
Yams	8 oz. serving	20	---	340
Bread, 25% flour	1 oz. slice	20	8	40
Peanut butter	32 gm (2 tbsp)	10	---	210
Rice	8 oz. serving	2	9	86
Banana	8 oz. (one)	11	95	770
Apple	8 oz. (one)	7	---	105
Strawberries	4 oz. serving	20	---	60
Peach	6 oz. (one)	9	---	196
Apricot	2 oz. (one)	5	---	100
Pineapple	6 oz. slice	15	---	138
Pumpkin	8 oz. serving	60	---	500
Grapes	5 oz. serving	10	---	140
Prunes	1 oz. (one)	10	---	210
Raisins	3 oz. serving	40	---	580
Recommended Daily Consumption (RDC)		**2500**	**1000**	**5000**

129

Note: 1) Most nutritionists consider these listed foods as healthful.
2) Values will vary somewhat from producer to producer.
3) RDCs are author's personal opinion (for average adult).

Table 8: Recommended Daily Supplement Program

pH	Calcium plus Magnesium		Vitamins D + A	
6.5 to 7.4 (healthy range)	1200 mg (3 tablets)	690 mg	2400 IU (6 tiny pills)	30000 IU
6.0 to 6.5 (developing a disease)	2400 mg (6 tablets)	1380 mg	4800 IU (12 tiny pills)	60000 IU
4.5 to 6.0 (you have a disease)	3600 mg (9 tablets)	2070 mg	7200 IU (18 tiny pills)	90000 IU

Note:

1)   Calcium plus magnesium tablets, sometimes referred to as dolomite, weigh 1400 milligrams (mg) and can be purchased in large retail stores, such as Walmart®, for about 2 cents each. Each tablet contains 400 milligrams of calcium and 230 milligrams of magnesium. Each tablet may also contain trace zinc, which is a bonus for your health.

2)   Consumption of magnesium in amounts greater than 700 milligrams daily may cause stool to become loose. If you are over this level, you will benefit from flushing the toxins out of your body.

3)   The tiny vitamin, A + D round tablet, or fish oil pills can also be purchased for just 2 cents each and contain 400 IUs of vitamin D, and 5,000 IUs of vitamin A.

For those of you that *just cannot take any more pills,* the author recommends that you crush and pulverize them into a powder and include them in your natural foods. For example, add to hot chocolate or cold fresh fruit juices for the elderly, or a milk shake for the kids. The author has found that the supplements taste good in both peanut butter and yogurt, but his personal favorite is to blend them with fresh fruit, such as cantaloupe, and ice in a high speed blender (*Vitamin-Fruit-Slush*). The author pulverizes a month's supply (25 tablets and capsules daily) containing every vitamin, all the essential amino acids, minerals that contain all of the essential major metals, such as calcium and magnesium, and every trace metal, including cesium and rubidium. The result is *one heaping teaspoon a day* added to a fruit slush.

The most frequent question the author is asked is, *"What do you do?"* The response always begins with, *"I have not taken a pill in over 30 years."* Psychologically, taking pills is synonymous with taking drugs. Also, many people have difficulty swallowing pills. For most, many of the pills remain intact as they pass through the intestine undigested. The obvious solution is to do what the author does. First, the author puts all of the non-liquid nutrient pills and capsules into a blender to make a pulverized blend. He then uses a flour sifter to remove the broken up oversized capsule containers. The author takes 24 pills and capsules each day, and he has found that when pulverized, the blend fills a heaping teaspoon. Thus, the author pulverizes a three-month portion and puts it into a large bottle labeled, *"Hunza Powder,"* and then takes a heaping spoonful each day. Second, the nutrient blend should be taken at meal times; for the elderly, this is the only time that they have sufficient acid in their stomachs to digest food. Third, one glass of milk or one glass of apple juice should be taken with each meal so that the lactates or malates will keep the digested nutrients ionized even as they pass through the alkali duodenum, thereby allowing for greater

131

absorption. Also, the consumption of fruits and vegetables with meals provides anions which enhance the absorption of nutrients.

The second most frequently asked question is, *"what are the 24 pills that you take?"* The answer is: 3 coral calcium (1.5 grams); 2 vitamin D (5,000 IUs each); 6 multivitamins (one-a-day); 6 multiminerals (containing 60 trace minerals); 3 calcium (citrate); 1 magnesium citrate; 2 vitamin C (60 mg each); 1 vitamin E (500 mg), and 10 milligrams cesium chloride. The result is *Hunza Powder*. The author takes a heaping teaspoon each day, usually mixed in a fruit slush or a banana shake.

One should remember that consumption of calcium as a supplement is like consuming dairy products, consuming magnesium is like consuming vegetables (magnesium in the chlorophyll is what makes plants green), and vitamins A+D like fruits, vegetables and liquid sunshine. Also, *vitamin D dramatically improves the absorption of nutrients by the small intestine.* Science has shown that, in the amounts recommended, these supplements cannot hurt you, but they can make all the difference to your health. Thus, Grandma was right when she said, *"The secret of good health is milk, fruits, vegetables and sunshine."*

Unfortunately, Grandma was only half right, as *when God made the Earth and all its inhabitants, he used all of the basic elements*, and most these basic elements are *sadly "missing" from our mineral-depleted soils* and thereby our food chain. The first humans had all of these elements in their bodies. The water that they drank and the fruits and vegetables they ate also contained all of these elements. The Biblical patriarchs lived to an astounding old age: *Adam lived for 930 years, Methuselah for 969 years and Noah for 950 years.* After the great flood covered their lands with nutrient-depleted sand and clay, the Biblical patriarchs did not live as long: *Eber lived to 464, while Issac only lived to 180 and Jacob to 147.* Today, except in rare areas of the world where degenerative disease does not exist and the average life expectancy is 135 years, the soils and therefore, the foods grown in them, are depleted of most of these minerals and *the life expectancy is 76 years.* The only exception are *American doctors who live for only an average of 58 years*, while the *average American*, who has a hard time following the doctor's nutritional advice, lives for *76 years.*

The *"common denominator"* of the many cultures, who live to be 135 years old while maintaining a vigorous youth in *disease-free* societies, is that *their soils are being constantly replenished with the mineral nutrients, most of which are missing in our soils.* Except for some of the Japanese on Okinawa, all these societies all live in mountainous regions. They are the Tibetans, the Hunzas of Northern Pakistan, the Armenian, the Georgians, the Azerbaijanis, the Vilcabamba Indians in Ecuador and the Titicacas in Peru, and a few other cultures. They all have their soils replenished with mineral nutrients contained in *the turbid water from melting glaciers.* The contained glacial-crushed minerals are so abundant that the water is white and is known as *"milk of the mountains."* The islands of Okinawa were built up over the years from coral reefs. Rain erodes the corral minerals producing mineral rich *"milk of the oceans."* All of these cultures also drink their water turbid. The contained dissolved minerals are so abundant that when they drink their customary two quarts each day, *"all"* of these disease-free societies *violate* our society's sacred Recommended Daily Allowances (RDAs) by massive amounts. For example, they consume *70 times* the RDA of calcium, *22 times* the RDA of magnesium, *18 times* the RDA of potassium, *126 times* the RDA of iron, *120 times* the RDA of fluoride, and so on. And, to top off these violations, they continue to exceed these RDAs even further by eating foods which are rich in these minerals. Also they consume *"RDA-unacceptable"* amounts of trace metals in their water while many maintain a diet rich in ingredients frowned on by Western medicine, such as *eggs, fat, milk, butter and salt*. The Hunzas drink their 30 daily cups of tea, each with a large hunk of rock salt and two patties of butter. Our American disease-ravished doctors, who die prematurely, ignorantly recommend that you *do not* follow the dietary example of the *youthful, energetic, and disease-free 135 year old Hunzas*. Nutrient-trained veterinarians, on the other hand, have long recognized the importance of mineral, metal and vitamin supplements, and as a result, animal foods are full of these supplements. For example, horse food and dog food can contain as much as *60 nutrient supplements*. Meanwhile, human food remains almost totally depleted in these life-sustaining nutrients. As long as the animals are fed only animal foods and not people food, they remain relatively disease-free.

Also of worthy of note is a product that has been consumed by the Japanese for hundreds of years with a huge number of health benefit claims; it is known as *"coral calcium,"* and is currently being consumed by increasingly large numbers of people in the Western world. Another product known as *"kelp calcium,"* has been consumed by Americans for the past 30 years. Both nutrients are mined from old ocean beds. When they are soaked in water, significant amounts of calcium, magnesium, and other trace metals are dissolved. What this means is that the minerals are already ionized before entering your stomach. This is especially beneficial to *the elderly* who increasingly, with time, *have less acid for digestion*. This, combined with the bicarbonate anions and the many microbes beneficial to absorption of nutrients by the body found in the coral calcium water, (*"milk of the ocean,"*) helps to keep the minerals *ionized longer* and therefore leads to greater mineral absorption by the body than most minerals consumed in other forms.

By now, despite the ignorant pleas from these doctors who go to their graves prematurely, you are probably wondering,

134

"Where can I get some of this *mountain milk water, or ocean milk water* or *sea milk water?*" The problem is that there is only enough mountain milk water to sustain a small number of people, and 100% of it is consumed. The more abundant ocean milk water is now available in America as *"coral calcium."* The sea milk water contains too much arsenic for the FDA and would thereby be outlawed. Unfortunately, having access to ocean milk water or sea milk water for drinking purposes will not solve the problem of mineral depleted fruits and vegetables. The only answer would be to *replenish our soils with all of the life-sustaining minerals and trace metals* and begin consuming them in the produced food. Also, mineral and metal nutrients could be added to the water supply. Many believe that the addition of trace lithium, for example, to our water supply would dramatically reduce mental disorders.

Table 9: Some Crucial Trace Metals

Metal	———————— Biochemical Purpose ————————
Boron	Needed in trace amounts for calcium uptake and healthy bones, and for the maintenance of normal levels of estrogen and testosterone in the blood.
Bismuth	Kills the bacterium **helicobacter pylori** which is proven to be the **"cause"** of peptic ulcers.
Chromium	Essential in manufacturing cholesterol, fats and protein, and maintains proper blood sugar levels and is therefore crucial in deterring diabetes.
Cesium	The largest and most alkaline metal, which, once inside the human cell, cannot leave, thereby neutralizing the acids which **"cause"** the degenerative diseases.

Table 9 Continued

Metal	———————— Biochemical Purpose ————————
Cobalt	Necessary for the production of the thyroid hormone, and is a crucial component of vitamin B-12, which helps prevent anemia.
Copper	An important component of hundreds of human enzymes, which help maintain the body's elasticity (youth), especially in the skin (preventing wrinkles) and in the cartilage and muscles and thus, helps to prevent aneurysms, arthritis, cerebral palsy, hernias, etc. Also restores color to graying hair and is crucial for iodine utilization.
Germanium	Acts as a carrier for oxygen, similar to hemoglobin, and is therefore excellent at tissue oxygenation to help prevent viral infections.
Iodine	Crucial component of the thyroid hormone thyroxin which regulates heart rate, body temperature, digestion, general metabolism, body weight, the nervous system and reproductive system.
Lithium	Helps to dissolve kidney stones. Helps to control criminal behavior and depression. Lithium deficiency can lead to manic depression, reproductive failure, and reduced growth rate.
Manganese	Crucial component of many hormones, enzymes and proteins and is an activator for cartilage and bone development. Manganese deficiency can lead to deafness, asthma, carpal tunnel syndrome and birth defects.

Table 9 Continued

Metal	——————— Biochemical Purpose ———————
Molybdenum	Constituent of many crucial enzymes including aldehyde oxidase, sulfite oxidase, and xanthine oxidase.
Praseodymium	Enhances the proliferation of normal cell growth, and in laboratory tests has **doubled the life span** of some species of animals.
Rubidium	The second largest and second most alkaline metal, which, once inside the human cell, cannot leave, thereby neutralizing the acids which **cause** the degenerative diseases such as cancer, heart disease, arthritis, etc.
Selenium	Selenium is the strongest metal antioxidant: it prevents cellular fats and lipids from going rancid and producing age spots and liver spots. It also helps to prevent heart palpitations, liver cirrhosis, sclerosis, cystic fibrosis muscular dystrophy, multiple sclerosis, Alzheimer's, cancer, etc.
Silicon	Silicon helps keep fingernails and hair from becoming brittle,while more than doubling the collagen in bone growth.
Tin	Helps prevent both hearing and hair loss while also helping to prevent cancer.
Vanadium	Enhances DNA synthesis and stimulates blood sugar oxidation, helping to prevent diabetes.

Table 9 Continued

Metal	———————— Biochemical Purpose ————————
Yttrium	Enhances the proliferation of normal cell growth, and in laboratory tests has **doubled the life span** of some species of animals.
Zinc	Required for protein synthesis and collagen formation, necessary for a healthy heart and healthy lungs, and promotes a healthy immune system and also promotes the healing of wounds.

However, this cannot happen overnight, and our health problems require immediate attention. Thus, until it happens, a manmade nutrient substitute with the right mixture of minerals, vitamins, and crucial trace metals (Table 9) will have to be provided. But this would be in violation of the laws in a society, such as America's, which suppresses nutritional therapy and where *medical freedom,* (the *right to choose* and the *right to practice* the medicine of your choice) *does not exist.*

The amounts of supplements in the *Recommended Daily Consumption* (RDC) substantially exceed the ridiculously low RDAs set by the establishment, as does the actual consumption by cultures free of degenerative diseases, and therefore, *will be "blindly" condemned by our medical establishment.* However, if God, or Hippocrates, the Father of Medicine, or your body were to be allowed to judge which is right, the RDCs found in the *milk of the mountains* and the *milk of the oceans* would be the clear-cut winner, *so claims the author!*

CHAPTER SEVENTEEN

CORAL CALCIUM AND MICROBES

In the beginning of time when life began in the ocean, one of the most primitive organisms was coral.

Coral reefs are formed over thousands of years with thousands of different corals. Some reefs build up into islands like Okinawa.

These reefs are gradually worn away by the waves and the weather. The ground up coral sinks to the seabed where it mingles with the water and its contained mineral and plant life.

Over millions of years the coral is biochemically altered to contain all of the mineral nutrients of the sea as well as its original nutrients of life. The result is a powerhouse of natural marine nutrients known around the world as,

"coral calcium."

The recently published book, *Barefoot on Coral Calcium: An Elixer of Life* by Bob Barefoot is the most comprehensive book ever written on coral calcium. It is published by *Pan American International Nutrition Publishing* or *phone 928-684-4458*. Of course, calcium plays an integral role in coral calcium, and the author suggests that once the reader has read this book and grasped the significance of the chemistry of calcium, he then read *Barefoot on Coral Calcium* so that he will also grasp the significance of the chemistry of coral calcium. This chapter can be considered a teaser for this great book.

Okinawa has the highest percentage of 100-year-olds in the world. What's more, your average Okinawan centenarian has the arteries of a child. A massive, ongoing, 25-year study has found that these 100-year-olds have 80% fewer heart attacks than Americans, and less than one-fourth the level of breast, ovarian and prostate cancer. Their younger brothers in their '80s and '90s seem to have the physical constitution of very young men and women. Five-hundred years ago, these features attracted the attention of the Spanish explorers who discovered the use of coral sands by these Okinawans. When the chickens would eat the coral sand, they would produce more delicious eggs. When the cows licked the reefs, they would produce more milk. The Okinawans also recorded 400% increases in rice crops when coral sand was used as a fertilizer. Because of the youthful and relatively disease-free culture, the Spanish filled their ship holds with the coral sand. Back in Spain, the chemists analyzed the coral and found the major ingredient to be calcium. The product was then referred to as coral calcium. The world's oldest drugstores in Spain, which are historic monuments, had their shelves lined with clay pots with the label, "Coral Calcium from Okinawa Japan." Today, the use of Okinawan coral calcium has spread to where millions of people in Japan, China, Russia, Sweden, and Europe are all taking the product daily. And the number of testimonials is staggering.

Of course, everyone is asking, "If Okinawan coral calcium is so good, what about Hawaiian coral calcium. The answer is that Okinawan coral is different from all other corals. The reason is that most coral reefs have significant wave action that washes the coral sands out to sea. Okinawa is a group of very shallow islands with virtually no wave action, and thus the coral sands build up to the point that they almost choke the reef to death. The government-supervised harvesting of the coral sands actually rejuvenates the reefs and brings them back to life. In addition, the Okinawan reefs are different in that numerous islands are of volcanic origin. This provides dramatic amounts of metal nutrients to the reefs. And lastly, Swedish scientists have identified marine microbes specific to Okinawa. Thus, millions of years of the coral reefs leaching the oceans have made the Okinawan coral calcium a treasure trove of nutrition, even though many of the nutrients in the ocean are found in trace quantities.

Gold, for example, is believed to be 0.012 parts per billion. This calculates out to be 460 billion ounces of gold or over 100 times the gold currently held in all the world's vaults. When gold is present in the soil, which is usually the case, it accumulates in the plant's protein and chlorophyll. The roots of plants can even break up rock, liberating the gold for uptake by the plants. When animals eat the plants, gold accumulates in the proteinaceous substances, such as hair, liver, brains and muscle. Man not only eats the bread made from the golden wheat, he also eats the animals that ate the gold. In many countries, gold leaf is popular in the diet. Gold is found in man's liver, brain and muscle, and human blood has been measured at 0.8 parts per billion, and 43 parts per billion have been found in human hair. Human feces and urine have been known to contain startling amounts of gold: the ash of human excretion has been known to contain one-third of an ounce per ton or over 10,000 parts per billion. The fact that gold exists in the human body in such significant amounts means that it must serve a useful function. Gold has been used successfully in some

141

cancer treatments. Gold suspended in gel has also been used to treat wounds, resulting in rapid recovery and minimized scaring. There are hundreds of industrial processes where gold is used as a catalyst, and one day man is certain to discover that gold serves as a crucial biological catalyst in the human body. Thus, the oceans are an enormous collection of metals, minerals and chemical substances that sustain life. The seas contain many factors that are produced by its own living organisms.

The coral calcium from Okinawa contains the perfect biological ratio of calcium to magnesium, 2:1 or 24% calcium and 12% magnesium. It also contains a host of trace metals. Coral calcium is a rich source of iron, containing almost 1,000 ppm. Next to calcium, iron is the most abundant mineral in the human body, crucial for maintaining oxygen. Iron permits effective oxygen transport and storage in muscles and the blood. It is the central component of hemoglobin in the red blood cells. Iron deficiency causes anemia and abnormal fat metabolism. Iron competes with other elements for absorption into the body (competition with magnesium, copper, calcium and zinc). Vitamin C enhances iron absorption and classic consequences of iron deficiency are weakness, fatigue, poor immune function and anemia. The common belief is that "too much iron can be toxic." The problem with this is that the words "too much" have never been defined. Also, United Nations Health Agency (UNESCO) says that the majority of American women are anemic, as a result of iron deficiency. Although the RDA for iron is 18 mg/day of iron, many nutritionists advocate at least 40 mg/day. The full-term infant requires 160 mg, and the premature 240 mg during the first year of life. The 240 mg at the average 5% absorption when consumed, equals 4,800 mg/year or 13 mg/day for the first year of life. The RDA for an adult is 18 mg/day. Also, for pregnant women, there is a requirement of 1 mg/day; at 5 mg/day this is 20 mg/day consumption. Pregnancy also increases demand for iron. Expansion of the mother's red blood cell mass requires 400 mg of iron, and the fetus and placenta require an additional 400 mg iron. Blood loss at delivery—including blood loss in the placenta—accounts for another 300 mg iron. The total requirement for a pregnancy, therefore requires about 1,100 mg iron. At 5% iron absorption, this works out to 90 mg/day consumption requirement for a pregnant woman, but the RDA for an adult is only 18 mg/day. Thus, most women in America are being poisoned by iron deficiency.

$\quad$**A** crucial factor in human health is that the human body is only capable of absorbing about ***800 milligrams of calcium each day***. Many of the calcium supplements are only in the 2 to 3% absorption range, while the so called *"great"* supplements are about only 15%. Cultures like the Hunzas, who consume over 100,000 mg of calcium each day obviously get their 800 mg absorption, while harmlessly passing the rest in their urine and excretion. With the Okinawans — because of the rod-like microbes in the coral, discovered by Swedish scientists in the 1990s — claim that the absorption approaches nearly 100%. Therefore, taking 250 mg of calcium in an antacid product, which does severe harm to the elderly by wiping out there crucial stomach acid supplies, usually results in the absorption of 5 mg (2%) calcium by the body over a 20-hour period. Also, there is substantial evidence that the nutrients in coral are ***absorbed in less than 20 minutes*** (the blood chemistry undergoes a drastic change, for the better, in less than 20 minutes). Therefore, the 250 mg of calcium in the coral results in 250 mg being absorbed by the body in less than 20 minutes, and without destroying the crucial stomach fluids. That's almost ***"50 times as much calcium, 50 times as fast."*** No wonder the coral calcium works so well! In addition, when people have major diseases, the consumption of a triple dose of coral provides the maximum calcium absorption.

$\quad$Coral calcium was first introduced to Western culture when it was brought to Europe by the Spanish explorers about

500 years ago. The world's oldest drugstores in Spain, which today are historic monuments, have clay pots on their shelves labeled "Coral Calcium, Okinawa, Japan." Literature written by doctors of the day told of miraculous cures. By the turn of the twentieth century, the consumption of coral had spread to mainland Japan, where currently there are millions of daily users worldwide. When coral calcium was brought to the Western communities as a "modern" dietary supplement in the 1970s, much misunderstanding was propagated by marketing companies. There is a naïve notion that when coral calcium is added to water it should dissolve completely. I am often asked about this circumstance, but the answer is obvious. If coral were soluble in water completely there would be no coral reefs in the oceans!

The reason why this question is asked often relates to the popular use of coral sand in tea bags which are merely added to water and the water is then consumed. Whilst coral calcium tea bags can import desirable properties to water, such as the transfer of important marine microbes, taking coral calcium in this manner is far less desirable than consuming the whole coral in powder or capsule form. Tea bag coral is less effective, as the user is only benefiting from about 2% of the marine nutrients that dissolve and the consumer – unless told – is almost unaware that he is consuming coral water. A more valuable way of obtaining the full benefits of coral calcium is consuming it in its complete format, resulting in the consumption of over 50 times as much mineral nutrients. Also, the marine coral that is totally consumed is rich in the required nutrient, magnesium, as well as richer in all other nutrients.

Fossilized coral that has been washed up onto beaches has lost some of its mineral content by weathering and it may be dried and finely powdered to make a quick change of water pH. In addition, some commercially available coral calcium products have calcium added in hydroxide forms to increase alkalinity. Also, fossilized coral contains less than 1% magnesium, whereas marine coral has about 12% magnesium, which balances the 24% calcium for a perfect biological 2:1 calcium/magnesium ratio. Because of this lack of magnesium in fossilized coral, magnesium compounds are often added, resulting in a substantial dilution of the coral. After studying many types of coral supplements, I have concluded that marine coral, not fossilized coral, taken in complete format is obviously the most ideal way to consume coral calcium for health.

Many commercial companies have promoted coral calcium from Okinawa as though it is all the same material. However, the harvesting of marine bed coral calcium is much more difficult and costly than merely collecting fossilized coral from beach mines. This fossilized coral has undergone thousands, if not millions, of years of erosion, losing most of its magnesium content and much of its trace metal nutrient content. Also, because of the hype generated by coral calcium testimonials, numerous, unscrupulous entrepreneurs are harvesting coral from other locations around the world (this coral does not have the desired microbes), but telling their customers that it comes from Okinawa. Some even go so far as to blend their coral with Okinawan coral so that they can make the claim that it comes from Okinawa.

Despite the deficiencies, both tea bag coral and fossilized coral consumption has led to remarkable health testimonials, although not as many as the consumption of marine coral. This is due to the "microbe factor" (explained in detail in the next paragraph). There are some who would believe that the microbes would be destroyed when the coral is heated for dehydration purposes. However, rod-like bacteria can survive poor conditions, such as severe drought, heat, radiation and various chemicals. They do this by forming structures called endospores. A single bacterium will form a small sphere-shaped or oval shaped spore within its cytoplasm. This endospore is protected by a tough outer covering. It remains dormant until favorable conditions reappear, when the spores develop into bacteria cells. In addition, there are many other factors that make coral calcium of marine origin more ideal for health. I prefer coral that is used in vegetable capsules or at least capsules that are made to dissolve at the right time to provide the best circumstances for mineral absorption. The practice of breaking capsules and adding the contents to water is unnecessary, except in circumstances where some people cannot readily swallow capsules

Microbes or bacillus are defined as any genus of rod-shaped bacteria that occur in chains, produce spores and are active only in the presence of oxygen and water. Although some microorganisms are destroyed in the process of drying, this process is not lethal to microorganisms per se. The addition of water can spring them back to life. Microbes can be found living in all living animals and plants. Of course most microbes can live off of plants and food, and are best known for their ability to "spoil" the food. Actually, spoiling food is a form of digestion. Thus, spoiled food is pre-digested by the microbes. This is probably the reason that most of the animal kingdom, including humans, has substantial numbers of microbes in their intestines. The strong acid in the stomach cannot break down all food, especially complex carbohydrates. However, the microbes in the intestine living off of these foods do indeed break them down and make them available for absorption by the small intestine. Also, the rod-like shape allows the microbes to penetrate deep into the "finger-like villi," five million lining the intestine, where they can easily be absorbed by *1) facilitated diffusion* (glucose combines with a carrier substance which is soluble in the lipid layer of the cell membrane), *2) osmosis* (the movement of water molecules and dissolved solids through semi-permeable cell membranes from an area of high concentration to an area of low concentration), *3) filtration* (movement of solvents and dissolved substances across semipermeable cell membranes by mechanical pressure, usually high pressure to low pressure), *4) dialysis* (separation of small molecules from large molecules by semi-permeable membrane) and *5) pinocytosis* (or "cell drinking" where the liquid nutrient attracted to the surface of the cell membrane is engulfed). As a result, the *"microbes are crucial to life."* Fortunately, most of the hundreds of non-marine microbes found in the human intestine were transferred by the mother. Some animals, like the baby elephant, have to eat their mother's excrement just to get the needed microbes.

The liver, pancreas, and intestine, all secrete fluids to assist the absorption of nutrients. Each day the liver secretes almost a quart of yellow, brownish, or olive-green liquid called bile. It has a pH of 7.6 to 8.6 and consists of water, bile salts, bile acids, a number of lipids, and two pigments called biliverdin and bilirubin. When red blood cells are broken down, iron, globin and bilirubin are released. The iron and globin are recycled, but some of the bilirubin is excreted into the bile ducts. Bilirubin is eventually broken down in the intestines, and its breakdown products give feces their color. Other substances found in bile aid in the digestion of fats by emulsifying them and are required for their absorption. Each day the pancreas produces about a quart and a half of a clear colorless liquid called pancreatic juice, which consists mostly of water, some salts, sodium bicarbonate and enzymes. The sodium bicarbonate gives the pancreatic juice an alkaline pH (7.1 to 8.2) that helps neutralize stomach acids and stops the action of pepsin from the stomach, and creates the proper environment for enzymes in the small intestine. The enzymes in the pancreatic juice include a carbohydrate-digesting enzyme, several protein-digesting enzymes, the only active fat-digesting enzyme, and a nucleic acid-digesting enzyme. The intestine itself produces up to three quarts of intestinal juice. It is a clear fluid with an alkaline pH of 7.6. It contains water, mucus, and enzymes that complete the digestion of carbohydrates, proteins and nucleic acid. Thus the liver, pancreas and intestinal juices are crucial in the digestive process, which helps to liberate the nutrients. Bacteria also play a crucial role in the digestive process as well as in the absorption process.

The genera of bacteria that are found in the intestinal tract are: Bacteroides (22 species, non-sporing rods), Clostidium (61 species, heat-resistant, spore-forming rods), Citrobacter (2 species, lactose-fermenting rods), Enterobacter (2 rods, ferment glucose and lactose), Escherichia (one specie, rods), Lactobacillus (27 species, non-sporing rods employed in the production of fermented milks), Proteus (5 species, aerobic rods that hydrolyze urea), Pseudomonas (29 species, most important bacteria in spoilage of meats, poultry, eggs and seafood), Salmonella (1,800 species that ferment sugars and glucose), Shigella (4 species, aerobic, like pollutuon), Staphylococcus (3 species, coagulate blood, also common in nasal cavities) and Streptococcus (21 species).

Salt greater than 1% can cross the cell membranes of most bacterium by osmosis, which results in growth inhibition and possibly death of the microbes. Everyone is also familiar with the preservation of meat by *"salting,"* which kills or inhibits the bacteria. Thus, large quantities of salt in the intestinal tract, which occur when large quantities of nutrients have been digested (hydrochloric acid from the stomach reacting with the sodium bicarbonate from the pancreas produces salt in the duodenum), can kill the microbes, thereby inhibiting nutrient absorption by the body, especially when large amounts of nutrients have been ingested.

On the contrary, *"marine microbes,"* such as those found in coral calcium by the Swedish, thrive in high-salt environments. Also, because of their original salty marine environment, as well as their calcium, magnesium and mineral environment, the marine microbes have no difficulty assisting the body in absorbing high quantities of these minerals, especially when the intestine is saline, resulting from the consumption of large amounts of mineral nutrients. These same salts, however, incapacitate the natural microbes in the intestinal tract, thereby inhibiting nutrient absorption. Thus, the coral marine microbes resolve this problem, dramatically increasing the absorption of the nutrients by the body.

Those people using a small sachet teabag that allows only a tiny amount of coral to dissolve in the liquid in which they are placed, and those using fossilized coral, still get some benefits from the marine microbes, hence the testimonials. Also, these testimonies emanating from the small intake of nutrients are nothing short of astounding. The reason for this success is that when the teabag or the fossilized coral is placed in a liquid, the microbes come to life and are consumed when the liquid is drunk. These microbes can then latch onto nutrients already in the duodenum and pull them into the body, resulting in health benefits. Consumption of marine coral, on the other hand, allows the *"total nutrient content of the coral"* to be consumed as well, and therefore provides far greater health benefits, leading to more testimonials. The bottom line is that all coral from Okinawa has fantastic health benefits, but the *marine coral is far superior*.

Coral is also very much like human bone, so the body does not reject it, and it is conducive to allowing new bone growth. In Germany, surgeons will pack the cracks and holes in the broken bones of the elderly with a coral paste made from coral calcium and water. Within three weeks the coral is displaced with new bone growth. James Tobin in *The Detroit News* writes that "because of a gift from the sea, coral calcium, Christian

Groth is swimming again. The coral rests snuggly inside the femur (thigh bone) of his right leg, just above the knee. It fills a hole the size of a large marble, replacing a benign tumor that was making it harder and harder for Chris, 14, to play the sports he loves. If you use a powerful microscope to compare the coral to Chris' bone, you could not tell the difference. Chris is one of the first people in Metro Detroit to have a bone repaired with sea coral and is 'doing everything,' said his doctor, Ronald Irwin, an orthopedic oncologist affiliated with the Beaumint Hospital, Royal Oak. 'It looks good,' Irwin said, 'he'll ski this year!'"

The May issue of *The New England Journal of Medicine* (2001) wrote about the "bionic thumb." Doctor Charles Vacanti at the University of Massachusetts recreated a thumb for Paul Murcia who had lost his thumb in a machine accident. First a small sample of bone from the patient's arm bone was cultured to multiply. Then, a sea coral scaffold was sculpted into the shape of the missing thumb bone, and then implanted into Murcia's thumb. The patient's own bone cells, grown in the lab, were then injected onto the scaffold. The bone cells grew a blood supply and the coral scaffold slowly melted away, leaving a new, living thumb bone. The doctors predict that eventually all that will be left will be a thumb bone with healthy bone cells and no coral. Twenty-eight months after the surgery, the patient is able to use his thumb relatively normally and the doctors say that the experiment in tissue engineering using the coral is working.

All testimonials are considered hearsay and are inadmissible to most scientists. However, when testimonials begin flooding out of countries all over the world, by sheer number, they themselves become scientific fact, and scientific fact cannot be ignored by any scientist. Although coral has only been in America for a few years, already the testimonies are flooding in. Here are a few examples:

TESTIMONIALS:

#1.   Hello, my name is Conrad Sims, I am 29 years old and I live in Decatur, Ohio. I am athletic and consider myself to be in good health. A few months ago, my neck began to get sore and then began to swell. I tried to ignore it, but it began to become painful. It was not long before the swelling was the size of a golf ball and my co-workers demanded that I see a doctor. It was diagnosed as malignant cancer and the doctor told me that it had to be removed surgically. He said there was no other way. I did not have health insurance for the surgery and I was terrified. A friend suggested I try coral calcium. I thought "what's a little calcium going to do for me?" I was desperate so I started taking the coral and within a week the pain had subsided. After two weeks the size of the tumor was dramatically reduced, and after four weeks it appeared to be gone. I am back to my old self and feeling great.

God bless coral calcium, Conrad Sim. (March 2001).

#2.   My name is Sue Ann Miller and I live in Akron, Ohio. I had been suffering for years with several diseases: diabetes, Bell's palsy, carpal tunnel syndrome, and I have had hip knee and elbow replacements. I lived on drugs and was in constant pain. I could barely walk and could not climb stairs. Then my sister went to a talk by Mr. Barefoot and brought me some coral calcium. I was in such pain and was so desperate that I would try anything. In just a few weeks the pain went away. A few weeks later and I returned to full mobility as my swelling went down and my hands straightened out. A few weeks more and I could bend over, touch my toes and run up stairs. I have gotten my life back. The coral was magic and I thank God for the coral and Bob Barefoot.

I love you all, Sue Ann Miller, Ohio.

#3.   My name is Donna Crow and I am struggling to recover from chronic fatigue syndrome which struck me severely 12 years ago. One of the problems with CFS victims, as I am sure you know, is that we have problems absorbing and/or using minerals. As a result we often have insomnia, heart palpitations and multitudes of intestinal problems.

A friend told me about coral calcium. She sent me a tape by Mr. Robert Barefoot. I was skeptical because someone else had sent me coral calcium that came in little tea bags and I had tried it with no noticeable benefit. But I value this friend's nutritional advice and out of honor for our friendship I listened to the tape. It was so educational. It opened up, for me, a whole new understanding of the need for calcium in the body. I loved the information and was determined to try some.

I got my first bottle and opened a cap and dumped it in my mouth, since I seem to absorb better when I do that and within two minutes I felt the most amazing things in my body. Peace would be the best word to describe it. And from that day on I never have had the stress in my chest I had, had for 12 years prior. And my digestion is wonderful now; no acid reflux anymore. And I have NO heart palpitations at all.

This product is more wonderful to me than I can say. Unless you have had constant heart stress and other calcium/magnesium-related problems long term, you cannot imagine how wonderful it is to go through a day without those problems. It is like getting out of prison.

I have all my friends and family on this stuff and they ALL love it for various reasons. That is the beauty of getting your mineral needs met. Your body will use them to do the unique repairs that you need. The body is so smart. If you give it the tools to work with it will literally work wonders for you.

Thank you for a product that has been like a miracle for me.

Donna Crow,Newport, OR.

#4. Hi to everyone,

Just wanted to let you all know that I've been using the Coral Calcium, and it is definitely helping me. I am especially excited over the fact that I am sleeping better. My usual night activity is frequent urination, getting up 6 to 8 times in a 8 hour period to use the bathroom, plus I wake up in pain all through the night. Since the very first night, I slept at least 4 hours straight before I had to relieve my bladder, then I took another calcium (not sure if it was necessary at that point) and slept like a baby another 4 hours. It's wonderful. This happens every night now. I have had such a sleep deficit for so long. Now some more good news: I have less pain. Oh Thank God! I have Fibromyalgia, and after years of disability due to such horrible, constant pain, a wheelchair, and a walker, I have hope of getting better, and I'm not so fatigued. To have any less pain is a miracle, and such a blessing. Now if I can start exercising and lose weight I will be so forever grateful to this product, and to Donna. Exercising makes Fibromyalgia worse, plus I have a back problem, a foot problem, and very weak legs. But somehow I know I'm going to keep getting better. THANKS to Donna for sharing this info. with me. I encourage you all to try it also. I've taken other calcium products, but never achieved these good results.

Bless you all,   Joanie O.

#5.   My name is Allen Jensen and I have battled high blood pressure for years and have been diagnosed with diabetes for three years. Medication has helped me more or less keep both "in check," but has done nothing to lower either the blood pressure or my blood sugar level. Then, in October 1997, I was diagnosed with Guillaine-Barre syndrome, a neurological disorder in which the nerves are destroyed by a "glitch" in the body's immune system. I lost a great deal of strength and dexterity in my hands, arms and legs. My active lifestyle of riding horses and a 30-

year career as a telephone installer/repair technician ended with no choice but to take early disability retirement. In mid-May 2000, I began taking coral calcium. Blood work showed a drastic improvement from tests in November 1999. My triglycerides improved from 1074 to 510, cholesterol from 380 to 210, and my blood sugar from 284 to 168. My doctor told me to "keep doing whatever you're doing." With daily use of the coral calcium I am confident that I will eventually be able to discontinue all of my medications. Coral calcium has virtually given me back the life I was beginning to believe I would not be able to enjoy again.

Allen Jenson, Breckenridge, Texas.

#6.   With nothing to lose, we started giving our crippled arthritic dog, Bandit, 2 coral calcium capsules every day, figuring that if an average person takes 2/day to fight serious illness, then Bandit, at about 43 pounds should take 2. She takes her capsules in peanut butter! That was July 1, 2000. Within just a day or two, she was eating again and walking out into the backyard and "using the facilities." Within a week she was walking normally. In 2 weeks she would actually "trot" out to the backyard, get on and off the couch, and come upstairs. By the end of 3 weeks she was actually playing "wrestling" with our 4-year-old dog, something she had not done in 2 years. Our veterinarian saw her and asked what we had done to create the "miracle." He bought some coral and said that he would be experimenting on some of his patients. By August, Bandit was like a new dog. She'll actually run now!

Bob Zacher, Memphis, Tennessee.

#7.   My name is Lisa Macintire and my 18-year-old cat. "Tootsie," 9 pounds, started limping about 2 1/2 years ago and

154

became very stiff-legged. She couldn't jump on things, like the washer where she eats. She obviously had arthritis and was getting worse. About 2 months ago I started giving her 2 capsules of coral calcium every day, and in less than 2 weeks, she stopped limping. I kept giving her 1 capsule each day after that. In less than a month she started jumping and climbing all over the furniture. A checkup by the vet showed her blood work, urine, etc. revealed no ill effects. The vet's words were, "She's in perfect shape." The only side effect Tootsie suffered was "feeling GREAT." This coral calcium is truly a miracle.

Lisa Macintire, Memphis, Tennessee.

#8.   I was diagnosed with multiple sclerosis in 1978, and along with the disease came excruciating pain. In 1986, a pump was surgically installed in my abdomen, which put morphine into my spinal fluid 24 hours a day, and brought me modest relief. Last year, after 9 times in the hospital and 8 surgeries someone introduced me to colloidal minerals, which began to turn my life around. When I heard about coral calcium I thought, "How is a calcium product going to help me?" Well, I tried it June 24, and it didn't take me long to realize that this was not the run of the mill calcium. About the first of July, I realized that I had no pain. For the first time in 19 years I had no pain and I could work 12 hours a day without stopping to lie down.

Earl Bailley, PhD, Doctor of Divinity, Ohio.

#9.   Hi, my name is Dorothy Boyer and I will be 80-years-old in June 2001. I have had problems at nighttime with my legs. They get a nervous feeling and I have to get up and stomp around the room to get it to stop and then retire again. It is quite tiring to have to do this every night. My daughter has tried to help me with many kinds of calcium and magnesium products, some quite expensive and none gave relief. Then she found Mr. Robert Barefoot's coral calcium and said, "Try this." And the very first night I slept through the night without any leg problems. That was several months ago and I haven't had any nighttime leg problems since starting the coral calcium.

Also I am very happy because I feel like I can think again. I have been very active mentally all my life and just in the last year I started to have trouble concentrating and staying focused. After just a few days on this coral calcium I felt like I could think again. I am very happy about that.

The biggest thing though is that I have a congestive enlarged heart and it doesn't take much for me to get a really rapid heartbeat. Just putting on a blouse in the morning would cause my heart to race and I would have to sit on the side of the bed and just calmly breathe until it passed. From the first day I took coral calcium, I have not had that again and that is the thing I am most happy about. It was very scary and it is nice to not be afraid every day.

Sincerely,
Dorothy Boyer, Newport, Oregon.

#10.   Your book did wonders for me. I had reached the point that joint pain was a part of my everyday life. Then, six weeks on coral calcium and I had become virtually pain-free. Now, one year later, I feel better than I have in eight or nine years. Now my only problem is making my family and friends believe that being healthy can be so easy.

Rick Whedbee, Covington, Georgia.

#11.   My husband Mark had painful heel spurs. He was advised to have surgery. He began taking coral calcium, 6 per day, and within 2 months he almost was pain-free. Within 3 months, all of the pain was gone and the doctors have advised that he no longer needs surgery. Coral was a miracle, as Mark's job has him working on his feet all day long.

Betty Gosda, Illinois.

#12.   My name is Patty and my husband was recently diagnosed with prostate cancer. My husband is 69-years-old, 6'6", and works 12 to 14 hours every day from 5 am to 5 pm and later. Rather than expose himself to the horror of conventional treatment, he began taking coral calcium. After 3 weeks, he had more x-rays and no cancer was found. Three weeks later, he went for a second opinion and had more extensive x-rays and once again, no cancer was found. God bless coral calcium.

Patty, Ponca City, Oklahoma.

#13.   First of all, I want to start off by telling you about my brother. Mr. Barefoot, you have spoken with my father several times about him. He has lung cancer. When it was detected, he had four lesions on his lung, one was the size of a peach seed. My Dad convinced my brother to take coral calcium. After 6 weeks when they ran another scan, 3 of the lesions were immeasurable; the big one had shrunk 60%. AMAZING!!!

Jeff Townsend, Kentucky.

#14.   Your website and research has truly been a blessing in my recovery of Hodgkin's Disease.

Denise Horick

#15.   Just want to take a moment to thank you for all your help. What coral calcium has done for me over a brief period is nothing short of profound. I can't remember any time in the last 29 years that I wasn't in substantial pain... that is until now. I have tried every pain remedy the orthodox medical community has in their arsenal, including narcotics, steroids, and antiinflammatories, just to name a few. Most of them did a great job of messing with my head, a feeling I literally hate, but did very little for the pain. I know almost nothing about the science behind this majestic mineral, coral calcium, I only know that it works. I have more energy, more range of motion, and less pain than I ever thought possible! I know that there was a time in my life that I was pain-free, I just couldn't remember how it felt until now. There are no words I can think of to adequately explain how much better I feel or what it means to me. Thank you so very much!

Best Regards, Gary T. Schilling.

#16.   I heard about your program from a lady who attended your meeting in Twin Falls this summer. My husband has a rare genetic disorder called Alpha I Antitrypsin, which is genetic emphysema that develops because the liver is not functioning properly, therefore, the lungs do not function properly either. He has been under a doctor's care for 9 years. After learning about your recommendations to help heal disease, my husband began taking the vitamins and the coral calcium and has been on the program for program for 7 weeks. He let go of his drugs and monthly prolastin infusion program. He is now very careful about what he eats. He feels better and better every day and has just let go of his inhaler. He has seen great improvement. I would love to speak to you and share this miracle unfolding before our very eyes. You are wonderful... thank you for your research and efforts.

Mary Wiggins.

#17.   I thank you for the confidence that you built for me. After being diagnosed with melanoma with no real hope for treatment if it were to reoccur, I felt devastated. My surgery was done at the Mayo Hospital in Rochester which is suppose to be "world-renown for its advancements in medicine," but that can't mean advancements in reference to the treatment of cancer!! I now feel a sense of security for which I thank you. In a world of chaos and pain due to surgery, I felt that I was "drowning" in a sense, and thank you, thank you, thank you, from the bottom of my heart and the hearts of my precious family in Minnesota. I have given your information to anyone who has felt the perils of ill health and you are indeed held in high admiration for your work and devotion to healing mankind!! YES for CORAL CALCIUM!!!

Marcy in Minnesota.

#18.   I can't believe how different I feel after taking coral calcium. I lived with constant pain in my heel for months. I could not jog because I could just barely walk. After taking coral calcium for two months, the pain is gone. I am back jogging. I would not have done this if had not been for you.

Thank you very much, Russ Tomin.

159

#19.   When one has been active all their life, it is impossible to understand the pain one suffers when the body is ravished by rheumatoid arthritis. Knowing that it was important to stay active, I enrolled in a fitness class. One of the activities involved lifting weights (20 pounds) with my legs. Due to the weakened condition of my legs, I tore a vital part of my knee. This sent me to the doctor and to physical therapy. When the pain did not go away, the doctor realized that the rheumatoid arthritis had taken over. I had been diagnosed 37 years prior with lymphedema which had caused fluid buildup in my legs. There was no known cure. The fluid must constantly be pumped out of my legs. This caused further damage and I no longer could have the fluid pumped out. I was in exacerbated pain now. Then I learned about coral calcium. Within two weeks I began to notice an appreciable decline in the arthritic pain. Within three months I became pain-free and I am off my walker. Also, the swelling had gone down in my mouth and I could use my dentures once again. Even my barber commented on how thick my hair had gotten. I am now "72-years young" after only 3 months on coral calcium. I can't wait to see what 3 years on coral calcium will accomplish. All I can say is, God bless all those who have made nutritional discoveries, especially coral calcium.

Willette Barbee, Plano, Texas.

#20.   The "Cancer Answer." The first week of March 2001, my stepfather was diagnosed with leukemia. They wanted to start chemotherapy right away. He asked for a 21-day delay so he could start a nutritional program with coral calcium In addition, Bob Barefoot recommended vitamin D and other minerals. On April 3, 2001, he went back to the doctors to run further tests on his condition. The doctors were amazed and totally baffled. They told him for reasons unexplained he doesn't need chemotherapy and that everything checked out normal. Hey folks, I thought Bob Barefoot had a screw loose when he claimed "coral calcium" could cure cancer. Turns out, he was right!

Jane and Sharon Gerding, Baker, LA.

#21.   My name is Susan Hedrik, age 49. I worked in a furniture factory carrying, stretching and cutting large rolls of cloth until it almost destroyed my body. I've had back surgery and suffered from a painful bone spur on my right thumb which two doctors told me would have to be removed by surgery. I also suffer from arthritis in my left leg. I was introduced to coral calcium and began taking it on January 27, 2001, and after 4 weeks MY BONE SPUR WAS GONE!!! I now can walk without a limp from the arthritis and no longer have to begin my mornings with a heating pad on my neck. For me, coral calcium is a MIRACLE!!!

Susan Hedrick, IR from Lincolnton, NC.

#22.   I have a 14-year-and-6-month old Dachshund named "Andrea, " suffering from arthritis in her hindquarters. She couldn't walk without falling over. She was unable to jump on a bed or the couch, even with the help of a foot stool I purchased coral calcium for Andrea and after 5 days she was becoming more active. After 8 days she was jumping on the couch, begging for treats and running and playing. Andrea not only returned to normal activity, she also lost six pounds. Coral calcium also helped her teeth. Since she only has half of her teeth, I used to break her dog biscuit in half so she could chew it. Now, she chomps it down whole. As for myself, I have chronic arthritis in my lower spine. After seeing what coral calcium did for Andrea, I began using coral calcium myself. After 4 days I no longer had to take my prescription drug "Relafen," which costs over $3.00 per pill (I was taking 2/day). I now am a firm believer in coral calcium as I have personally witnessed what it can do.

Jack Polhill from Lincolnton, NC.

#23.   I would like to confirm that the use of coral calcium has been beneficial to my health. My knee replacements are deferred and my golf swing has improved. I'll be 74 this summer and I trust this sophomoric feeling is not second childhood.

Eugene T. Hall, Calgary, Canada.

#24.   I am an osteopathic physician practicing osteopathic manipulation in the cranial field in South Central PA. I have a patient who has suffered from severe fibromyalgia for the past several years. Recently she started taking coral calcium. This patient has improved dramatically. She has more flexibility and motion in her muscles and joints than she has in several years and she is nearly pain-free on many days. She has been able to continue a multitude of other medication, including chronic pain pills. The information in your books and tapes corresponds well to the science, the practical, the safe, the reasonable. I thank you for the time you have expended educating us.

Marianne Herr-Paul, D.O.

#25.   My mother, who has been on coral calcium for the past two months, paid a visit to her doctor to have her cholesterol

162

retested. Her cholesterol had dropped 204 points and the doctor was amazed! She is now a believer in coral calcium. I thank God for you finding this product that is changing people's lives and giving their health back.

Cindy Metzger.

#26.   My cousin Shirley had been diagnosed in May with breast cancer and colon cancer. She was scheduled for a double mastectomy and was also going to have her colon removed. You advised her to take the coral calcium and other nutrients and by July the breast cancer was gone and the colon cancer had shrunk. (**Note:** The October 1, 1998 issue of *Annals of Internal Medicine* printed a Harvard study of 89,000 women that found daily multivitamins reduced the risk of colon cancer by as much as 75%). Her doctors, needless to say, are absolutely amazed. I can't thank you enough for helping my cousin, Shirley, as she means everything to me.

Patti Hernandez, Oklahoma City, Oklahoma.

#27.   I am 62-years-old and have always enjoyed good health. In July 1997 I was diagnosed with *prostate cancer*. The diagnosis was confirmed with a biopsy and an ultrasound. Two of six biopsies were positive with cancer. My doctors strongly urged me to take hormones and have my prostate removed. I thought about it but looked for alternative remedies. For six months I boiled Chinese herbs and did Qui Gong exercises and thought that this kept the cancer in abeyance. But in the spring of 1998 a second biopsy turned out to be similar to the first. As a result of reading *The Calcium Factor*, I received excellent treatment and eventually cured myself of prostate cancer. A third biopsy in July 1998 showed only one positive but reduced active cancer. I

163

continued to take coral calcium and other supplements. A fourth biopsy in January 1999 showed that where the tumors had been, there was now only benign prostatic tissue. I had beaten the cancer. As a result, I would strongly recommend that anyone suffering from cancer or similar debilitating diseases, should study Barefoot's book, *The Calcium Factor,* and take responsibility for their own health. I have yet to find anyone who has written such well-reasoned and scientifically based material. I have been taking coral calcium for 3 years and it has saved my life.

David G McLean, Chairman of the Board, Canadian National Railways.

#28.   In October 1996 I was diagnosed with *prostate cancer.* The diagnosis was confirmed by biopsy. In October of that year I started following Robert Barefoot's coral calcium regime. In July 1997 I had another prostate biopsy in which no evidence of malignancy was found. The regime outlined in the book, *The Calcium Factor,* improves the immune system to where the body can heal itself, without intrusive measures like surgery, chemotherapy or radiation.

S. Ross Johnson, Retired President of Prudential Insurance Company of America.

#29   I am a physician, President and Executive Medical Director of Health Insight, S.B.S. and Health Advocate Inc., in the state of Michigan. I have extensive credentials and honors that reach the White House and heads of states in other countries. Mr. Robert Barefoot has worked over the past 20 years with many medical doctors and scientists across the United States and in other countries doing orthomolecular research on various diseases. The information has been culminated in the book, *The Calcium*

Factor, which has been used technically as a Bible of nutrition. Many people I know have thanked Mr. Barefoot for *both saving their lives and returning them to good health*. Mr. Barefoot is an amazing and extraordinary man who is on a "great mission" for all mankind. I thank God for Robert Barefoot and thank God for coral calcium.

Liska M. Cooper, M.D., Detroit, Michigan.

#30.   Mr. Barefoot has been, and continues to be, an advocate for health and natural healing through nutrition and knowledge. He has championed the cause of well over 440,000 American women and children who have been exposed to the *toxic effects of silicone-implanted devices*. Mr. Barefoot, one of the rare silica chemists in the world, has delivered a message of hope to these suffering individuals, who didn't have any hope before, but are now arming themselves with the book, *The Calcium Factor,* and are spreading the word, especially about the miracle nutrient, coral calcium. His work with hundreds of scientists and medical doctors researching diet has elevated him to be one of the top speakers on nutrition in the nation.

Jill M. Wood, President Idaho Breast Implant Information Group, Boise, Idaho.

#31.   I graduated from Harvard University in 1942 (BScChemistry) and worked as a research director and in corporate management, and have been awarded two patents. Mr. Barefoot has been highly influential in my survival of *prostate cancer*, with which I was diagnosed in the fall of 1991. Because of his detailed knowledge of biochemistry, he has much more penetrating knowledge of the relationship between disease and nutrition, a knowledge not available to many trained dieticians

165

because of their lack of biochemical background. With his expertise, he has aided me in not only arresting the progression of my disease, cancer, through diet and nutrition with coral calcium, but also reversing it.

Philip Sharples, President Sharples Industries Inc. Tubac, Arizona.

#32.   I am a chemist and have been involved in product development, specifically nutritional supplements. I have written numerous articles and lectured throughout the United States on these products, especially coral calcium, and the benefits of utilizing alternative medicine and alternative medical products within the U.S. healthcare regimen. Over the past three years, I have traveled and lectured with Mr. Barefoot on numerous occasions all over the United States. He is recognized as a world-class expert on calcium, especially coral calcium, and its nutritional benefits for the human body. I have personally seen Mr. Barefoot's information help a lot of people.

Alex Nobles, Executive Vice President, Benchmark USA, Inc., Salt Lake.

#33.   One year ago, my son Tim had **major back surgery**. Several discs had been crushed and three surgeries were performed. Four discs were removed, part of his hip bone was removed and ground to mix with a fusing material, then four cadaver knee cap bones were put into areas where the discs were removed. He has two titanium rods, two cross braces and eight screws in his spine. He started on coral calcium the day after the surgery. The first follow-up doctor's appointment showed that the fusion was doing great, exceeding the doctor's expectations. He said that this surgery was one of the toughest cases he has had. He

166

said that he was amazed with the results, and told us to keep doing what we were doing. When Tim ran out of coral calcium for 3 or 4 days, he complained of severe back pain, which disappeared as soon as he went back on the coral calcium.

Billyr J. Stein, Ponca City, Oklahoma.

#34.   The meeting that I had with you changed my life and how I think about my health. I am the person whose cousin's wife you helped. She took your coral calcium and minerals and she no longer has a *brain tumor*. My cousin's name is Gary Elias and his wife's name is Diane Elias. They live in Woodbury, Connecticut and they are both grateful because Diane's brain tumor pretty much dissolved and has not returned.

David Querim, Connecticut.

#35.   In November 1999 I was diagnosed with *prostate cancer*. My PSA was 244!!! On the way home, I listened to your audio tape. Talk about having the hand of God in your life!!! I knew in my heart that this is what I should do. Once I started, I never deviated from the plan. The results were amazing after only one month!!! My PSA had dropped to 25.5. By May, my PSA was 4.6 and I had my doctor and specialists scratching their heads over my instant recovery. My doctor said that he never expected me to live past the end of January 2000. We also prayed and my doctor told me that "maybe the prayer worked," but it could not have been the calcium and supplements. Fortunately, others have listened. My brother-in-law no longer has *high blood pressure*, ulcers, or indigestion. His sister-in-law no longer gets *cramps in her legs* and her *arthritis* is getting better. Her 5-year-old grandson, who suffered so much from *leg cramps*, no longer has pain or cramping and he can sleep all night long. These are just a few stories.

Bob Heinrich, Keremeos, British Columbia.

#36.   Video *The Calcium Factor*, with numerous video testimonials, 800-443-9935.

CHAPTER EIGHTEEN

CARL J. REICH, M.D.

No story on the state of Western medicine today would be complete without describing a living example of what it is like to be a doctor struggling within the system to serve his patients with technology rebuked by the system, but supported by science. To even be allowed to do this, the process has to be gradual and not too offensive. Then, if public support is attained, after silent shunning by your peers, followed by verbal sniping from behind, and ending with sarcastic acceptance of you as a *living example of a "quack,"* you may be allowed to continue your practice of medicine. But, except for a few doctors like Carl Reich, this is rarely allowed. No doctor is allowed to challenge the financial base of medicine, and unfortunately, this was the crime that caused Dr. Reich to lose his license in 1983. He believed that degenerative diseases, such as cancer, arthritis, heart disease and even AIDS could be cured and prevented by doctors addressing the nutritional deficiencies of their patients. His only mistake was making representations of his proposals to the government. The medical *judge-jury-prosecutor system* moved swiftly to invoke their *"preordained"* **guilty-by-daring-to-challenge-the-system verdict**. What Dr. Reich did not understand was that, regardless of his high moral motives and his real concern for public health, medicine cannot be changed without first changing the system, and therein lies the real crime, as Dr. Reich had so much more to contribute to human health.

Dr. Carl J. Reich was a product of one of the most orthodox and rigid medical systems in human history, and yet, he chose to defy the system to provide his patients with the therapy which, from his clinical research on other patients, he knew would provide them with the best health benefits. That constituted practice, which 30 years later would be identified as preventive alternative medicine. As he began his practice in 1950, Dr. Reich began clinical research by applying the benefits of the discoveries he had made in his post graduate studies in internal medicine. Almost from day one, he was known and shunned as a medical maverick who chose to practice *contrary to current medical opinion.* By 1954, his clinical research led him to conclude that most of his diseased patients had led a lifestyle that rendered them deficient in one or both of calcium and vitamin D. He scoured the medical literature seeking guidance, but without much luck. Had he scoured the scientific literature (science almost always precedes medicine by several decades) he would have had much more luck as science was beginning to give biochemical calcium a high position in importance to human health. Unaware of this, Dr. Reich had to fight the *medical battle of ignorance* alone, at least in the beginning.

When Carl Reich was a young man, his Austrian immigrant father from Vienna died of cancer at the age of sixty-two. Carl had always known his father to be a sickly man, plagued from childhood with constipation, obesity, and in his later years, with severe migraine. Of course, everyone knew that a son is likely to follow in the footsteps of his father, but Carl was determined not to do this. As a result, he chose to live a different lifestyle than his father, who never exposed his hands, face or arms to sunshine, and the most nutritious food that his father ate was his annual two glasses of buttermilk. Early in his life, Carl, living in the small northern fishing village of Prince Rupert, British Columbia, was fed white bread, macaroni, canned vegetables, meat, sugar and syrup with a dash of canned milk in his coffee.

The result was a life full of colds, constipation, cramps and boils. When Carl was 12, in order to save money, he persuaded his father to stop purchasing expensive meat and to only eat the inexpensive fish. The result was the beginning of his disease-free years. Carl resolved to eat as much nutritous food as possible: all the fruits and vegetables he could find and gallons of milk. Sunbathing also became a familiar regiment, as Carl *took to the hills,* hiking the mountains while stripped to the waist, a practice that he still continues to this day, and he is approaching 80 years old. The result was that Carl, unlike his father, who never knew good health and what it was like to live without pain, lived a very healthy life.

In 1938, Carl became a medical student and in 1940, enlisted in the army, where he continued his studies. After serving in Canada, England and Germany during World War II, during which time Carl's health had suffered from the lack of nutrition during wartime; Carl began four years of postgraduate training in internal medicine. During these early years the benefits and toxicity of megavitamins were being researched and debated. Because Carl was enjoying personal health undreamed of by his father, Carl knew that it was because of nutrition and a healthy lifestyle. He therefore, unlike most of his contemporaries, became indoctrinated into the belief that ailments should be prevented and not treated. Lifestyle meant exposure to certain dietary and environmental factors that promoted good health, while avoiding foods that inhibited good health. Carl wanted more definition of these factors.

Thus, it was not surprising to find Carl, in his final post-graduate year, researching the injection of drugs, such as adrenalin, that stimulate the functions of all organs of the body. The drugs produced different blood pressure responses that contemporary medicine attributed to stress. But, because of Carl's nutrition background, he believed that the responses were attributable to *different levels of mineral deficiencies.* Carl

171

reasoned that, since much disease was attributable to imbalanced excitation, caused by mineral deficiency of the body's organs, identification of these imbalances in an apparently healthy person with no symptoms of disease could be used to predict the occurrence of impending disease. He became determined to assess these imbalances by analyzing large numbers of patients for different symptoms and physical changes that were believed to cause these symptoms.

From the beginning of Dr. Reich's medical practice, he immediately began to recognize that many of the medical ailments about which his patients were complaining were accompanied by what he suspected was mineral deficiency, particularly calcium, accompanied by a lack of exposure to sunshine. During this research, in one decisive week in 1954, Dr. Reich treated four of his patients, whom he had studied and determined to be calcium deficient, with intravenous injections of calcium. These patients were experiencing one or more of the diseases of chronic diarrhea, chronic asthma, constipation, leg cramps, rhinitis, and nasal sinusitis. He followed the calcium injections with calcium gluconate, and vitamin D-rich halibut liver oil, taken by mouth. The results were an astounding resolution of all of the symptoms and diseases. He then concluded that these lung and intestinal diseases were not caused by *allergic reactions*, as modern medicine had thought, but rather were caused by reactions created by *calcium mineral deficiency*. He reasoned that ionic calcium had relieved the smooth muscle spasm and reduced the secretion of mucous in both the lung and small intestine. Spurred on by these successes, he then treated a seven-year-old boy, who had been suffering from chronic asthma since birth, with only oral calcium, vitamin A and vitamin D capsules, and was happily amazed to find that *the asthma was **almost completely relieved** – and in just **three days***. Furthermore, the asthma never reoccurred as long as the child remained on the supplements.

By giving his patients mineral and vitamin supplements, and by recommending – just as Hippocrates had recommended to his patients – healthy changes in lifestyle, such as exposure to lots of sunshine and fresh air, he was able to turn their lives around, many claiming miraculous cures. As word of his success grew, his practice flourished. He tried in vain to share the fruits of his success with his medical peers and friends, but they reacted by shunning him as if he had the plague. They just could not understand *how something so simple could have any merit*, which was the same argument that prevented doctors from washing their hands for so many years. Meanwhile, Dr. Reich became extremely frustrated that the patients of his blind and deaf medical peers continued to suffer and die from the same ailments, which he was able to cure in his patients. The matter was further aggravated by both the way in which Dr. Reich's medical practice flourished, invoking professional jealousy, and by the way Dr. Reich resisted the arbitrary restrictions imposed by medical committees, boards and councils.

At this time in medical history, *stress*, such as infection, trauma, starvation, worry, and overwork, was believed to trigger disease. It was thought that exhaustion of the adrenalin adaptive system, which produces the hormones that regulate metabolism and muscular energy, resulted in what was then known as *adaptive diseases*. However, the pattern emerging from Dr. Reich's clinical studies confirmed that stress could not play a decisive role unless the adaptive system was already compromised by mineral deficiency.

In 1958, after observing and treating thousands of patients, Dr. Reich concluded that chronic disease, such as asthma, ileitis, and colitis were not the direct effect of *ionic calcium deficiency* on the lung and intestinal tract, but rather, by a breakdown in the adaptive function of the body's organs attempting to compensate

173

for the deficiency. Thus, he regarded heart disease as *asthma of the heart*, and colitis as *asthma of the intestinal tract*. He therefore began to successfully treat these diseases with calcium and vitamin D supplements. He concluded that most degenerative diseases resulted from calcium and vitamin D deficiency and defined his concept as a *"unified concept of disease"* based on those deficiencies. By now, Dr. Reich was known to all of his peers as a medical maverick.

By the 1960s, Carl Reich had caught up with science and science had caught up with Carl Reich. In the Max Planck Institute in Berlin, where Dr. Otto Warburg, Nobel Prize winner, had proven that *cancer was anaerobic* (a condition, such as acidosis, where the body fluids lack oxygen), Carl presented his thesis that the cancer cell was not absolutely anoxic, but only functionally anoxic due to calcium deficiency, and therefore could not utilize the oxygen in its environment. Carl went on to find that the cancer in many of his patients seemed to go into remission once their calcium deficiency was rectified by a change of lifestyle, accompanied by mineral and vitamin supplements. Their associated mineral deficiency diseases were also suppressed.

By 1972, *Dr. Reich had discovered that the saliva pH reflected the mineral deficiency*, and therefore the *state of disease* of his patients. He continued to document this co-relationship on thousands of patients. Again, this test was treated with a chorus from the medical establishment of, *"How could something so simple have any merit?"* No wonder Dr. Reich became so frustrated.

In 1983, one year after the new HIV viral disease had been described as *acquired immune deficiency syndrome (AIDS)*, Dr. Reich suggested that this disease may represent both immune and *adaptive deficiency*. He therefore coined the syndrome

"*AAIDS*" to more correctly describe the disease. Dr. Reich began presenting his theories to leaders in the research and therapy of AIDS, where there was stiff competition for the megabucks research could bring, as well as government leaders. His proposal was to correlate the lifestyles, the mineral deficiency and the saliva pH of healthy athletes, HIV virus carriers, and AIDS patients. This proposal would be very inexpensive to execute, and could have resulted in *stopping AIDS in its tracks*, as those who carried the virus may have demonstrated that they could not get the disease, AIDS, as long as they did not become mineral deficient. Thus AIDS, one of the most *financially lucrative diseases* for the drug and medical industries, could have been stopped before it took hold of America. Within months of this proposal, Carl J. Reich, M.D., medical pioneer, had his license to practice medicine suspended.

Thus, while the orthodox doctor today both cures and kills with the brutally painful procedures of the twentieth century, Dr. Carl J. Reich, and others like him, cure with the painless procedures of the twenty-first century, as no patient was ever killed by implementing a healthy change of lifestyle, including a diet supported by moderate supplements of vitamins and minerals. The result, in Dr. Carl Reich's case, was over 20,000 satisfied patients with a much improved state of health. Many of these patients were the children whom Carl adored, and most of whom responded to treatment within days. Their allergies disappeared or were dramatically reduced, and those who were labeled as unmanageable quickly became the leaders in their classrooms. The elderly also benefited as many crippled with arthritis became well again. Dr. Reich's success rate was very impressive and very self-satisfying.

In the September/October Issue of *City Scope*, a well-read magazine in Calgary, Canada—the city where Dr. Carl Reich practiced medicine—a feature article, "**Ahead of His Time,**" was published as a tribute to his pioneering efforts with preventive medicine. The article refers to Dr. Reich as the *"father of preventive medicine,"* and gives him the **main credit** for having Bill 209, known as the Medical Profession Amendment Act, passed in the Province of Alberta Legislature. The bill simply states: *"A registered practitioner shall not be found guilty of unbecoming conduct or found to be incapable or unfit to practice medicine or osteopathy, solely on the basis that the registered (practitioner) employs a therapy that is non-traditional or departs from the prevailing medical practices, unless it can be demonstrated that the therapy has a safety risk for that patient unreasonably greater than the prevailing treatment."* Thus, for the first time in North America, a government has put the **burden of medical proof on the accuser**. Unfortunately, although Dr. Reich took pride in the bill's passage, he noted that *"these Doctors know what's in the best interest of their careers, even if it's not in **the best interest of their patients.**"* When Barefoot took Reich his first copy of the magazine, Reich responded that *"unfortunately, although the article is extremely flattering, it was written **ten years too late** for me because I'm getting much too old to really take advantage of the new law."* Two months later, ***Dr. Carl Reich, the father of preventive medicine***, passed away in his sleep.

Unfortunately, with the orthodox approach to medicine, degenerative disease is rampant, and we are not only losing the wars against these diseases, we are also losing the brave pioneering soldiers who are fighting the battles to court-martials by their jealous generals. There is an argument that innovators are not products of the system, but rather innovators are born into the system. Either way, the result is the rare and unusual individual who is forced to challenge the existing system, which is always based on self-preservation. If America hopes to turn the tide against disease, the dreamers must prevail.

"Some men see things as they are and ask why? Other men dream of things that never were and ask why not?" (President John F. Kennedy)

CHAPTER NINETEEN

VITAMIN D AND BLACK AMERICA

Every once in a while the newspaper will write an article on just how sick Black America is with a specific particular disease. When all of the articles are collected, however, a much different story appears. *Black America almost has twice the cancer* (American Cancer Society, "Cancer Facts and Figures for Americans 2004-2005.") *Blacks have 60% more cancer and 250% higher death rate than Whites; twice the diabetes and five times the kidney disease; and even more tragically, life expectancy for Black men is 68.6 years old compared to 75.0 for White men (6.4-year difference) and for Black women it is 75.5 versus 80.2 for White women (4.7-year difference)* (American Cancer Society, "Cancer Facts and Figures for Americans 2004-2005.") This is a *six-year* discrepancy for men, and almost a *5-year* discrepancy for women that makes me want to scream!!! I am very angry that the medical authorities can stand by and let this happen. In my life, I have never seen a worse form of racial prejudice. It makes me sick and ashamed to live in America. It is definitely *the crime of the century.* Black America is dramatically sicker than White America and dying much younger. *Why??? Why??? Why???*

Why??? Please, Oprah Winfrey and Jesse Jackson help me stop this injustice!!!

And why don't the medical authorities do something about this absolutely disgraceful situation? And, why don't White Americans even know about it? And why aren't the Blacks talking about it? Unfortunately, the answers lie in our ignorance and the medical authorities who are leading us. In 100 years of trying, they have not been able to inhibit or cure even one disease, not one!!! These generals of medicine have been leading us in a war against disease where they have lost every battle. And then, when they win a little skirmish, they make sure that they get credit and it is given front page headlines. The reason that they are losing this war, where all of our lives are pending – including those of our children – is that they are looking for a white chemical drug to answer their prayers. This is just never going to happen.

If we are to survive as a nation, or even survive as a species, we must replace these ignorant generals of medicine in the AMA, FDA and FTC with the men of vision who understand that the answer lies in nutrition. If I were given charge of these organizations, I would fire the incompetent generals and revamp these organizations to make them serve the public, which is what Congress intended when it created them. There would be dozens of FDA-approved medical claims for calcium and vitamin D and the FTC would stop harassing nutritionists who would now be FDA-approved. The FDA would actually assess food and preventive medicine so it could then become the medicine of the twenty-first century. *"If the doctors of today do not become the nutritionists of tomorrow then the nutritionists of today will become the doctors of tomorrow."* – Rockefeller Institute of Medical Research, New York.

Thus, there is hope on the horizon, as medical researchers all over the world are finding that supplementation with the humble mineral calcium, along with vitamin D, can help to prevent and even cure disease. Thus, it may soon be possible to cure America, but in fairness, and with God, we must cure Black America first.

Before this can happen, we must understand the reason why Black America is so sick. The answer lies on the beaches and at the swimming pools of America, for there you will find Caucasians in bikinis and bathing suits, lapping up the sun and producing vitamin D, inisitol triphosphate, calcitonin, melatonin, serotonin and a whole bunch of other "tonins." The sun on the skin produces crucial enzymes that regulate mineral disposition in the body. The sun is necessary for good health. While Caucasians flock to these public sunbathing locations, the Black community avoids the sun like the plague, and in doing so, cuts itself off from crucial biological functions, such as the production of vitamin D, and they are thereby being ravaged with disease and dying young.

The sun striking the eyes causes the glands behind them – the pituitary, pineal and hypothymus – to produce the hormones calcitonin, melatonin and serotonin along with others. Thus, the sun-avoiding Black community does not produce the enzymes, hormones and vitamins that are crucial to good health and hence, they are twice as sick as the White community. The first step to good health for the Black community is daily exposure to God's sunlight and the health benefits that it provides.

Unfortunately, there is a further complication with the Black community and the sun. It is a natural sunscreen called melanin, that evolved to protect humans from blistering solar radiation as they evolved in equatorial regions of the world. This skin pigment is an extremely effective sunscreen, with absorption properties from the ultraviolet into the visible range. Thus, people of color, who have greater amounts of melanin in their epidermis than do Whites, are less efficient in producing vitamin D than are Whites. Because of the darkness of their skin and the different content of melanin, Blacks require *10 to 50* times the exposure as whites to produce the same quantity of vitamin D (**"Vitamin D: Importance in the Prevention of Cancers, Type 1 Diabetes, Heart Disease, and Osteoporosis,** *"* from the "Vitamin D Skin and Bone Research Laboratory" section of *Endocrinology, Diabetes and Nutrition*, Department of Medicine, Boston University School of Medicine, Boston. MA.) Thus, a White man sunbathing for 15 minutes produces more vitamin D than a Black man sunbathing all day long. This basically means that regardless of the exposure to sun, Blacks will require vitamin D supplementation.

Who is Usually Deficient in Vitamin D?

In a recent study, Gregory A. Plotnikoff, M.D. of the University of Minnesota Medical School found that all of the African Americans, East Africans, Hispanics, and Native Americans who participated in the study were vitamin D deficient, as were all of the patients under the age of 30. The findings are reported in the December 2004 issue of the journal, *Mayo Clinic Proceedings*.

What Diseases Have Been Implicated
Due to Vitamin D Deficiency?

Alcoholism
Anxiety
Arthritis
Autoimmune diseases
Birth defects
Bone diseases
Bone pain
Burning in mouth
Cancer: prostate, colon, and
breast
Celiac-Sprue
Coeliac
Crohn's
Chronic fatigue syndrome
Chronic pain
Cystic fibrosis
Depression
Diabetes
Diarrhea
Enzymatic diseases
Fatigue
Fibromyalgia
Graves' disease
Heart disease
Hernia
High blood pressure

Impaired wound healing
Inflammatory bowel disease
Insomnia
Intestine
Irritability
Joint pain
Kidney
Liver
Lupus
Malabsorption
Multiple sclerosis
Muscle pain
Myopia
Nervousness
Obsessive disorders
Osteomalacea
Osteoporosis
Panic attacks
Parkinson's disease
Psoriasis
Rheumatoid arthritis
Rickets
Scalp sweating
Schizophrenia
Thyroid

*** To review more clinical studies, perform an internet search for "vitamin D deficiency" and the conditions listed above.

It is also important to note that everyone should avoid wearing glasses as they interfere with light striking the eyes which is crucial for hormone production. Also, avoid skin blocks because they interfere with biological functions. It is highly probable that in the near future there will be multi-billion dollar lawsuits concerning these matters.

Of course, for good health and longevity, a program of calcium and vitamin D supplementation will be mandatory. Marine coral calcium from Okinawa, Japan is the preferred form of calcium supplementation, the problem being that most of the coral calcium produced in America is not marine; it is fossilized or dirt coral, as it is dug out of the ground and costs a small fraction of the cost of high-grade marine coral harvested from the sea. Despite this, you will probably be charged high grade prices for the low-grade coral and it may even be in a bottle with the Barefoot label. If it is, you will usually be charged less, but you should be aware that the reason for the dirt cheap pricing is because it really is dirt. Unfortunately, surfing the Web for Bob or Robert Barefoot will result in about 2 million hits, which means that there is an enormous amount of knock-off coral on the market today.

CHAPTER TWENTY

THE FINAL CHAPTER IN MEDICINE

The layperson, having read this book, and therefore, having been exposed to constant historical conflicts between medical researchers and their governing establishments, may be confused as to what to believe and what to do. Many – especially the elderly – will rush to their doctors for guidance and advice. The author recommends that everyone do just that, as to many, the doctor is God. Doctors delivered us into life, attended to our ills since birth, and the doctor's advice, when incapacity or mortality threatens, is an absolute essential. The doctor is, and always will be, *the most respected member of our society.*

Unfortunately, because of the lack of medical freedom, the doctor's scope of knowledge on preventive medicine has been restricted by the governing establishment to the point where, although he may have opinions and concerns for your best interest, in reality he has no knowledgeable answers. For example, past experience has shown that the misinformed doctor may suggest that you could end up with a "massive kidney failure from all those pills." This, of course, is totally incorrect and misleading. It has been scientifically proven that nutritional supplements will do just the opposite, saving your kidney from failure. The term **"pill"** is also incorrect and misleading. Although many vitamin and mineral supplements can be purchased in tablet form, they are also natural nutrients (food) that are now available in many of the delicious products sold in health stores. The term **"pill"** refers to the unnatural chemical compounds being produced by drug companies who currently have everyone taking so many pills that almost everyone believes that they "just can't assimilate any more pills." Other misinformed doctors may even tell you that *vitamin D is toxic*, despite the fact that for decades, doctors prescribed drugs whose major active ingredient was vitamin D. The doctor is just passing on misinformation given to him by the medical establishment which, despite all of the scientific studies extolling the value of vitamin D consumption, really believes what it is saying. Thus, before you go to your doctor, the author also recommends that you first go to your local library to look up and verify the scientific and historical information provided in this book, so that, together, you and your doctor can discuss facts, and not just biased opinions based on misinformation.

Many others, especially the younger generation who, as Max Plank would say, "Will *finally change the system when the old die off*," will choose not to go to the doctor. They will, however, research the literature for verification of the astonishing facts presented in this book. Unfortunately, by not going to their doctor, they are missing their opportunity to express their opinion and to let the doctor know why most Americans are currently vying for alternative medicine. It is also a fact that there are more and more doctors who are getting away from conventional medicine, and actually practicing preventive and homeopathic medicine without being expelled from their associations, which are currently busy trying to legislate the public back to orthodox medicine. However, as history has taught us, if these maverick doctors are deemed to be a threat to the system, their licenses will quickly be revoked. Thus, change is definitely occurring and we are slowly chipping away at the managed medical mountain. But, we are being endangered by the *pending avalanche of legislation* which is being sponsored by the giant multinational drug companies. Unfortunately, the crises is about to become even worse. In April 1996, Congress passed, and the President signed innate law, the **Health Insurance Bill**. The bill contained a rider from the ***World Health Organization Codex Program*** that seeks to harmonize the governing and manufacturing of health and medical products, according to the standards set by the United Nations. The rider quietly passed. ***The Codex Commission Committee*** (90% of the Codex delegates represent giant multinational pharmaceutical corporations who are concerned about the ***potential encroachment*** of vitamins and minerals into their marketplace) has proposed the following guidelines for dietary supplements:

1.   *No dietary supplement can be sold for preventive use or therapeutic use.*
2.   *No dietary supplement sold as food can exceed the potency levels set by the commission.*
3.   *Codex regulations for dietary supplements would become binding.*
4.   *All new dietary supplements would automatically be banned unless they go through the Codex approval process.*

What this means is that, as of April 1997, the Food and Drug Administration has the authority to close down all health food stores and will require a medical doctor's prescription for vitamins, herbs and other supplements. Thus, the doctors with ***almost no nutritional education*** will be forced to participate, as the drug companies eliminate their only competition – nutritional health – thereby maintaining the current trend in America of ***disease out of control***. The result will be ***legislated disease***. In Norway, where similar legislation was passed, the result has been the closure of over half of the health food stores with the remaining in jeopardy. The average American, **62%** of whom have chosen alternative medicine (according to a recent televised poll by the Columbia Broadcasting System, commonly referred to as the CBS), will soon wake up to find that their choice of nutritional products has been removed from the market. The war against disease will continue to be lost and the average American will suffer enormous physical and financial pain. This is *"America's wake up call."* Only medical freedom enshrined in the Constitution can blast away all of the *mountain of ignorance and indifference*, thereby clearing the way for the preventive medicine of the twenty first century. Until this happens, legislation, similar to the Alberta Government's Bill 209, should be drafted and passed into law in America. This would at least force the drug-sponsored AMA/FDA partnership to *"demonstrate that nutritional therapy has a safety risk that is unreasonably greater than the prevailing orthodox medical treatment."* Of course, as history has constantly demonstrated, this is almost impossible to do when employing a *"scientific basis"* for the demonstration. For the sake of the health of America, the legislation should be *reversed*, forcing the drug companies to demonstrate that the safety risk for using their drugs is not unreasonably greater than the prevailing nutrient treatment. If this were to happen, *over 90% of the drugs currently sold by the pill mill would be removed from the market.*

The fear that the *doctor's job* may be in jeopardy when preventive medicine becomes established, which may needlessly be having some impact on the establishment's position not to support preventive medicine through nutrition, cannot be justified by the facts. Although there is little doubt that hundreds of billions of dollars and numerous prestigious empires are at stake, the average doctor need not fear change, as the ingenuity to survive always prevails. Besides, change will definitely come sooner or later, and the fears that change will cause the demise of the whole system have never been shown to be true. For example, television was supposed to have sounded the death knell of the movie industry, and yet today, it is the movie industry that is saving television. Another, and more appropriate example, is the effect that fluoridation of water – a form of preventive medicine – had on the dentists. I remember listening with amusement as the dentists of one city with un-fluoridated water complained that their counterparts in a nearby fluoridated city were *making more money* than they were making. The *experts* had predicted that a drop in cavity rates would result in a drop in the dentists' income, and as history teaches, *experts are rarely right*. As it turned out, people without cavities do not mind spending money on dental cosmetics, which is financially more lucrative for the dentists.

Likewise, there is no doubt that a society with a much-improved state of health from today's society, will also concern itself with more cosmetic medicine. The reduction of disease will result in the demise of some of the most expensive drugs, which will most certainly be replaced by nutrient supplement packages being dispensed from the very popular and busy doctors' offices. The drug companies will have most assuredly used their current massive profits to buy and reshape the *new nutrient industry*. Doctors will remain the most trusted and respected members of society.

In the late 1990s, an interesting trend began to immerge. The drug industry has begun to buy up the nutrient industry. Tens of billions of dollars have been spent already, and the rate of investment is growing rapidly. In late 1999, the vitamin industry was fined over one billion dollars by Washington for price fixing, to which they admitted. Interestingly, all of the guilty vitamin companies were owned by the drug industry. At the current rate of investment, the whole nutrient industry will be owned by the drug industry within a decade. Why is this happening? Perhaps the drug industry has had a wake up call. Although they can control medicine and the media in America, the world is a big place. In Russia, for example, doctors are reading *The Calcium Factor*, and are following through by prescribing vitamins and minerals to their patients with startling results. Apparently, Russians are curing cancer in Moscow using American know-how. It is only a matter of time before television will expose the results to the American public, and just as television brought down communism, television will also bring down the AMA and the FDA. That is, unless they don't *"discover"* nutrition first. Regardless, it appears that they will own it anyways, and if history repeats itself, the public should be prepared for some hefty hikes in the price of their nutrients.

In the near future, the healthy public will be griping about the new high cost of nutrients, while enjoying a temporary reduction in taxes brought about by the effect preventive medicine would have on dramatically lowering America's deficit. Thus, everything will remain the same, but, with *one* exception, the *death-by- diet-cycle will finally be broken.*

THE AFTERWORD

After detailing many of the misdeeds of the medical and scientific establishments over the past three centuries, as well as the litany of some of the world's most famous scientists speaking out against these establishments, the reader may be left with the impression that the problems of scientific advancement are the fault of these establishments. Although, indirectly, that may seem to be the case, in reality, it is not. The men and women who run these establishments were born into the positions. The system was there long before they came along. All they did was participate, and for doing so, were rewarded with positions of power, perks and prestige. The irony is that most of these men and women are people of high moral standards who actually believe in what they are doing. But, as history has shown, when human suffering prevails because of an archaic system, intentions are not good enough.

Great spirits have always encountered violent opposition from mediocre minds." (Albert Einstein)

The goal of good health for the masses will not be easy, as the ***undercover dictatorship*** referred to in 1776 by ***Dr. Benjamin Rush***, America's first Surgeon General and the only American doctor to sign the Declaration of Independence, is now

189

well-entrenched in the power structure and has its vested interest in continuing *to oppose* preventive medicine. Thus, the freedom *to choose* and the freedom *to practice* the medicine of your choice must be "*put back into*" the American Constitution. Dr. Benjamin Rush tried strenuously, but failed, to have "*medical freedom*" enshrined in the Constitution. He proclaimed that, "*The Constitution of this Republic should make special provisions for medical freedom,*" and that "*to restrict the art of healing to one class of men and deny equal privileges to others will constitute the bastille of medical science.*" He further declared that, "*All such laws are despotic and un-American.*"

The self-appointed protectors of your personal health will continue to stomp out medical competition and medical progress in the name of medical quackery. The computerized press makes it difficult for them to continue to do so, but a constitutional amendment, such as the following, putting back into the Constitution what was taken out at the last minute, enshrining Dr. Benjamin Rush's *freedom of medicine* as an equal to *freedom of religion,* would make it impossible for anyone to ever again impede medical progress, with the consequence being "*good health for the masses.*"

Each and every American citizen has the right to choose and to practice the form of medicine that the citizen deems most beneficial to personal health, without economic, physical, political, or verbal interference or abuse, and any institution or governmental agency assigned to protect the state of the individual's health should be empowered only to make recommendations that do not infringe or prevent the individual's right to choose and to practice any form of medicine.

However, amendments to the Constitution are very rare, and require years to succeed. The American public is desperate today, and cannot wait for this desperately needed change. Thus, the best interim remedy would be for each state to legislate an Alternative Medicine Protection Act:

"A practitioner of traditional or alternative medicine, registered by an appropriate government authority, who engages in medical or nutritional therapy or in any relevant health procedure, including the recommendation or sale of health supplements, that departs from orthodox or conventional medical treatment, shall not be found to be unqualified, unprofessional, negligent nor guilty of assault upon a patient, nor be denied the right to pursue her or his professional practice or livelihood, solely on the basis that the therapy employed is an alternative remedy, or is non-traditional or departs prevailing orthodox medical treatment, unless it can be conclusively demonstrated that the therapy has a safety risk for a particular patient unreasonably greater than the traditional or prevailing treatment usually employed for the patient's ailment."

Howard W. Pollock, Former Territorial Chairman of the Legislative Committee on Statehood for Alaska, and First Republican U.S. Congressman for Alaska.)

This would put a speedy end to the ***death-by-diet*** situation in which America now finds itself.

Death by Diet   by R. Barefoot

We are what we eat, and we are what we don't,
When told what to eat, some of us won't,
Cause to eat butter and eggs and milk and salt,
We are told will bring life, to a crashing halt.

And yet the cultures that do, they don't have disease,
They eat all of these things, as much as they please,
One hundred times the Recommended Daily Allowance,
Exceeding the RDA by the pound, and not by the ounce.

And every element, God put on the good Earth,
Is consumed every day, for its nutritional worth,
And they also eat lots of vitamins and lots of minerals,
Garlic and onions, they're not young at their funerals.

Lots of butter and salt, at one hundred having tea,
Americans we don't, and we barely make seventy,
All day in the sun with their lives is the trend,
Hippocrates was right, the sun's your best friend.

Yet these cultures have taught us "its not what we eat,"
But that which we don't, without nutrition we're beat.
We grow old while we're young, with premature death,
Believing we're right, as we exhale our last breath.

This premature death caused by doctor's advice,
Should cause the world to pause, and start to think twice,
With drugs so expensive, and vitamins so thrifty,
The shame is your doctor ages n'aire over fifty.

Drugs are man-made powders, chemicals that kill,
Vitamins and minerals, are God's design, his will,
And the health of the world, will be filled with sorrow,
If the doctors today, don't become nutritionists tomorrow.

Order Form

Web Site: "barefootscureamerica.com"
Toll Free 866-723-2551

Name:_____

Address:_____

_____

Country/Zip:_____

Phone Number:_____

Yes, I / We would like to order more copies of *Barefoot on Coral Calcium - An Elixir of Life* or *Let's Cure Humanity* or *The Calcium Factor* or *Death By Diet.*

Please send___copies of_____.

@ $24.95 US each ($27.00 Canadian)

for a total of $_____.___

Please allow a shipping and handling

charge of 5.00 US ($7.00 Canadian) per book: $_____.___

Arizona residents please add appropriate tax: $_____.___

Total enclosed: $_____.___

(Please check addition carefully; incorrect totals will be returned unfufilled.)

Please allow 2 to 6 weeks for delivery.

A quantity discount schedule is available upon request.

Mail this order form (or a copy) along with a check for the total amount to:

Complete Fulfillment & Distribution
P.O. Box 71058 | Phoenix, AZ 85050-1058, USA